THE YOGA SUTRAS OF MAHARISHI PATANJALI

Translated by
Yogachariya Jnandev Giri

ISBN 978-1-9995850-3-7

First Published March 2019

Imprint - Yogachariya Jnandev

Designed, Printed & Published by Design Marque

Printed in Great Britain by www.designmarque.co.uk

Foreword

The Yoga Sutras are important for all serious Yoga Aspirants to study, these sutras (verses) contain timeless wisdom that can help us to navigate our way through samsara (our experience of the world) and ultimately find some inner peace. I hope these pages can encourage us to keep reflecting on the true meaning of our life and the many paths of yoga sadhana (disciplined practice) that Yogamaharishi Patanajli reveals to us as a way to Moksha (ultimate freedom).

This work on Yoga Sutras of Maharishi Patanjali is my simple contemplative translation in my own understanding. There are many translations and commentaries on Yoga Sutras. Some of them are beautiful linguistic translations while others are scholarly work. This work is outcome of my Yoga Sadhana and studies of following works-

Yoga Step By Step by Dr Swami Gitananda Giriji.
Ashtanga Yoga by Dr Swami Gitananda Giriji.
Yoga Darshan by Dr Ananda Balayogi Bhavanani
Raja Yoga by Swami Vivekananda.
Yoga Sutras – A simple translation by Yukteshwarananda.
Yoga Darshan By Gita Press Gorakhapur.
Swamij.com, by Swami Rama.

This work is blessings and guidance of my Guru Dr Ananda Balayogi Bhavanani, Ammaji Meenakshi Devi and Dr Swamiji Gitananda Giriji, who have guided me on this path of Yoga as a life style and holistic path to health, well-being and self-realisation. I recommend all sincere yoga Sadhakas to come and experience true yoga under guidance of these true masters of yoga at Ananda Ashram (International Centre for Yoga Education and Research), Puducherry, India. I am also very grateful to Samaniji Sthitha Prajna Ji, who guided me on this path of yoga at a very beginning of my journey at Jain Vishwa Bharati, Ladnun.

I am also grateful to Yogacharini Deepika Saini and our three beautiful young yogis (Siddha, Mahadev and Krishna) who has helped me on this path of yoga since they have been part of my life.

With thanks to our designer Sarah Ray (Design Marque), who brings these writings forward for readers. I would also like to express my gratitude towards all my sincere yoga students who have always helped me grow through their enquiring mind and profound interest in learning holistic yoga and yoga sutras.

Content List

Blessings from Dr Yogachariya Ananda Balayogi Bhavanani 5

One must approach the yoga sutras with reverence,
by Dr Yogachariya Ananda Balayogi Bhavanani 7

Maharishi Patanjali Compiler of Yoga Philosophy 11

Four Chapters on Yoga 13

The Sanskrit Alphabet 15

Chapter :1 Samādhi Pāda 17

Chapter 2: Sādhanā Pāda 45

Chapter 3 : Vibhuti Pāda 75

Chapter 4 : Kaivalya Pāda 105

Blessings

Yogachariya Jnandev (Surender Saini) and Yogacharini Deepika (Sally Saini) are an integral part of my Gitananda Yoga family worldwide and I am so proud of the way they have been able to develop through hard work the Yoga Satsanga Ashram in Carmartenshire, Wales and well as their new International Ashram developing in Portugal. Having visited their Ashram in Wales, I can vouch for the beautiful spiritual ambience that can be felt there and it is a joy to teach in such a Yogic atmosphere.

May the Guru Parampara continue to bless Yogachariya Jnandev, Yogacharini Deepika and their family as well as the Yoga family of the Ashram with success in their Yoga Sadhana.

The yoga tradition is pan-universal and para-universal in its perspective. In this ancient art and science of right living, reverence is one of the most important qualities required in any sincere aspirant. Without reverence it is difficult to value "that" which we have and "that" which we have been given. It is difficult to understand how blessed we are if we choose not to realize it. The shat darshan are not just mere, philosophical perspectives of the dynamic universe but are a reverential witnessing of the Divine Universal Nature.

All aspects of yoga are sacred, not in a limited religious sense but in an unlimited spiritual one. All aspects of yoga need to be respected. It is only when we have such an attitude of respectful love, profound interest, that we can become a yoga bhakta. Then, and then only, will we be fit for these teachings of the highest nature.

Any attempt to explore the Yoga Sutra of Maharishi Patañjali must spring from an attitude of respect, reverence and love for these teachings. If that is absent, then one may as well as be reading any common magazine or newspaper instead. The place, the time and the frame of mind will enable us to develop the right attitude, the universal beatitude towards these elevating teachings. This reverence would be completely lost if we choose to treat them like other mundane information or data.

What attitude will you choose? The choice you make determines whether or not the treasure house of the Yoga Sutra opens its doors to you or not!

May we all grow and glow in spirit through the life of Yoga, enabling each and every one to manifest their inherent divinity with joy, health and wellness.

Om Hari Om tat Sat Om.

Yogacharya Dr Ananda Balayogi Bhavanani

MBBS, MD(AM), C-IAYT, DSc (Yoga)

Director and Professor of Yoga Therapy, CYTER of Sri Balaji Vidyapeeth and Chairman ICYER at Ananda Ashram, Pondicherry, India. www.icyer.com

ONE MUST APPROACH THE YOGA SUTRAS WITH REVERENCE

Yogacharya Dr Ananda Balayogi Bhavanani

MBBS, MD(AM), C-IAYT, DSc (Yoga)

Director and Professor of Yoga Therapy, CYTER of Sri Balaji Vidyapeeth and Chairman ICYER at Ananda Ashram, Pondicherry, India. www.icyer.com

One of the greatest minds of human history is the sage Maharishi Patanjali, the codifier of the Yoga Darshana (a reverential view of the highest reality through the art and science of Yoga). He must have been indeed an amazing man, for he is credited with giving us: Yoga for the purification of the mind (as Patanjali); Grammar for the purification of our language and speech (as Panini); and Ayurveda (ancient Indian medicine) for purification of the gross physical body (as Charaka).

It boggles our mind to even contemplate this great humane being who lived only for the welfare and spiritual growth of his fellow brethren. Patanjali was surely an enlightened soul who had experienced the highest state and yet stayed back because he wanted others to also have that Darshan of the Divine and attain the ultimate goal of "Kaivalya".

The eternal concepts of the Yoga Darshana have been codified in a nutshell through his Yoga Sutras. These Sutras must have been composed and then transmitted by the oral tradition since at least 1000 – 1500 BC but came into the written form much later in around 500 BC – 300 AD that is the commonly quoted date for them.

The Patanjala Yoga Sutra consists of short succinct Sutras that run together as if they were making up a garland of pearls on a string. This unique method common to the oral tradition of Yoga helps us grasp the intricacies of Yoga, this greatest science of inner experience that has been defined by Yogamaharishi Dr. Swami Gitananda Giri as the 'mother of all sciences'. The Sutras were always kept short as they were intended to be learnt, memorized and chanted with reverence and understanding in order to facilitate the development of a deep sense of quiet, inner contemplation. The Yoga Sutras are an efficient tool to help the sincere Sadhaka remember and understand the subtleties of the great art and science of Yoga and were NEVER meant to be a mere instruction manual.

All of the limbs of Maharishi Pathanjali's Ashtanga Yoga as well as Kriya Yoga have only the purpose of assisting the individual to grow towards the ultimate goal of Yoga, which is Kaivalya (liberation). As we gradually grow into the higher states of consciousness, there occurs the dawning of higher discrimination (Vivekanimnam), and when this occurs, the mind begins to gravitate towards absolute liberation from all experiences that otherwise result because of the interaction between the perceiver and the perceived. It is as if we are pulled into that highest state once we get close to it though our self-efforts!

As Dharma Megha Samadhi finally manifests, the Kleshas and Karma are removed once and for all by this potent rain cloud of virtue that has the potential to bless us with eternal freedom. The torrential rainfall from this rain cloud of the highest nature washes away all the arrogant, ignorant impurities that were keeping us away from our attaining to the highest state of ultimate realization. It is at this point that Maharishi Patanjali implies that we become the Divine itself in the state of Kaivalya as he had earlier defined Purusha as a special soul who is beyond Kleshas and Karmas. We become the Divine by losing our sense of individuality in order to gain the sense of absolute universality.

Once this state occurs, the Gunas automatically recede back into their essence having fulfilled their purpose of giving us both the enjoyment (Bhoga) as well as having stimulated us towards the attainment of emancipation (Apavarga). In fact, we actually even go beyond time itself (Akala) at this point. There is no more any ramifications of the past or the future for they disappear completely. At this point we finally exist totally only in the enlightened Now!

Patanjali concludes his teachings in the Kaivalya Pada by saying that once we reach this point in our spiritual journey, the Pure Consciousness becomes established in its own True Nature. With the attainment of this absolute and most dynamic state of being, our evolutionary journey ends, as we have reached the pinnacle by attaining to our true essence where division of any kind ceases to exist anymore. Indian philosophical thought tells us over and over, again and again that our essential, true nature is Sat-Chit-Anandam (Absolute reality-consciousness and bliss).

Maharishi Patanjali has given us an amazing and crystal-clear road map towards Kaivalya though his Sutras. Yet the onus lies entirely upon us to follow it with the twin keys of Abhyasa and

Vairagya for that is the only way that we can finally attain our goal of absolute liberation - once and for all. It is important that we never forget to remember his warning that we must Not Stop when the Siddhis appear for they are mere milestones on the path and must continue onward on our evolutionary journey from that of a mere human to the ultimate Divine.

I offer my deepest heartfelt salutation to the great Maharishi Patanjali, the incarnation of the thousand headed Adishesha. May he bless us all in our spiritual search for that highest state of Kaivalya!

Yogacharya Dr Ananda Balayogi Bhavanani

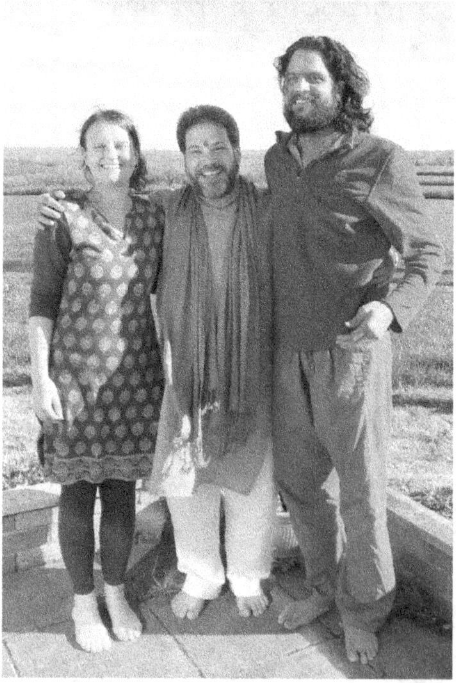

pictured here (left to right) Yogacharini Deepika, Yogachariya Dr Ananda Bhavanani and Yogachariya Jnandev Giri at Yoga Satsanaga Ashram Wales, UK.

Maharishi Patanjali
Compiler of Yoga Philosophy

About Maharishi Patanjali

It is believed that Maharishi Patanjali is the Avatar/incarnation of Adi Shesha - the Infinite Cosmic Serpent upon whom Lord Vishnu rests. He is considered to be the compiler of the Yoga Sutras, along with being the author of a commentary on Panini's Ashtadhyayi, known as Mahabhasya. He is also supposed to be the writer of a work on the ancient Indian medicine system, Ayurveda. The life history of Patanjali is full of legends and contradictions. There are no authentic records regarding his birth. According to one legend, he fell ('pata') into the hands ('anjali') of a woman praying for a child, thus giving him the name 'Patanjali'. In this story he was a baby snake being carried by a bird through the air and at the moment of the woman's prayer the snake fell from the bird into her palms. The story goes that she was dejected at this moment and as a great devotee of Shiva she wept with grief, so Shiva appeared before her and said "I cannot change what has happened but I can transform this snake into half man and he will attain my knowledge of Yoga". Hence Patanjali was born.

Another legend about Patanjali:

Adi Shesha found it unbearable to support the weight of Lord Vishnu, while watching a dance by Lord Shiva. Amazed at this, he asked Lord Vishnu the reason why this was the case. Lord Vishnu said that this was because of his harmony with Lord Shiva's energy state, owing to the practice of Yoga. Realising the value and benefits of Yoga, Adi Shesha decided to be born amongst humans as 'Patanjali', to teach them the great art and science of Yoga.

Patanjali's Yoga Sutras

The Yoga Sutras are considered to serve as the foundation of all yogic techniques. Maharishi Patanjali, also widely known as the father of Yoga, compiled 195 sutras, which serve as a framework for integrating Yoga into a daily routine and leading an ethical life. The exact date of the compilation of the Yoga Sutras is not known. However, it is believed that they were written somewhere around 2000 BC. The core of Patanjali's teachings lie in the 'Ashta-anga' or eight-fold limbs of yoga. The path shows the way to live a better life through yoga.

This practical system attempts to understand the nature of the mind; it's different states of being, the impediments to spiritual growth, it's afflictions and the methods of refining and stilling the mind in order to attain 'Samādhi', which means absolute bliss, deep joy, oneness with the super-consciousness. The central doctrine of Yoga philosophy is that nothing exists beyond the mind and its consciousness, which is the only ultimate reality. The objective of this philosophy is to uproot misconceptions about the existence of external realities from the minds of men/women. It is believed that it is possible to reach this stage of self-realisation through regular practice of certain yogic meditative processes, which culminate in complete withdrawal and detachment from all false sources of knowledge. This inculcates an inner sense of balanced calm and tranquility.

Four Chapters on Yoga

The Yoga *Sutras* begin with *Samadhi Pada,* which describes what yoga is; followed by Sadhana Pada; and then *Vibhuti Pada,* describing the benefits of yoga; and *Kaivalya Pada,* explaining the concept of absolute liberation or freedom from the cycle of birth and death.

Samadhi Pada (Union, Perfect Concentration)

Samadhi Pada is the first chapter of Yoga Sutras by Patanjali. He begins this chapter by defining yoga as a path of discipline and goal as Samadhi or Self-Realisation. In this chapter Patanjali deals with various states of mind, whirlpools of the mind and their outcomes. This chapter deals with all the mental issues we all need to deal with. Further Patanjali provides us tools to deal with these mental and emotional whirlpools or ups and downs. Further Patanjali details all the obstacles we have to deal with in our day to day life on this yogic evolutionary journey with also detailing all the tools we need to overcome these obstacles. Also Patanjali details various levels or types of Samadhi or Absolute Concentration and Union.

Sadhana Pada (Practice, Ashtanga Yoga)

Sadhana Pada begins with describing Kriya yoga (yoga of action), which includes Tapas, Swadhyaya and Isvara Pranidhanani. Patanjali explains that Kriya Yoga will help us to be free from all the sufferings of Karma, mind-manipulation, fluctuations and desires. Further Patanjali details The Eight Limbs of Yoga, or the eight-fold path (Ashta-anga yoga).

The eight limbs are-

Yama (restrains)
Niyama (observances)
Asana (posture, pose or seat)
Pranayama (subtle energy work)
Pratyahara (sensory withdrawl)
Dharana (concentration)
Dhyana (meditation)
Samadhi (Union or self-realisation)

Vibhuti Pada (Siddhis or Fruits of Sadhana or Yoga Practice)

Vibhuti has several meanings: It means fruits, blessings or outcomes of sincere Sadhana and Practice. Vibhuti also denotes the sacred ash that remains from the Yajna or fire ceremonies in Yoga Hindu Ashrams, which represents the purest form of blessing to bring health and well-being.

The Vibhuti Pada details begin with further detail of the inner limbs of Yoga (Antaranga Yoga) Dharna, Dhyana, and Samadhi. It details the benefits and fruits of Samayama or Higher Yoga in regard to various Dharna or Concentration practices. Vibhuti Pada gives us many concentration practices. This chapter also mentions the importance of going through repetition of all limbs of yoga and explains concentration, meditation and Absolute Union as integrated practices in the form of Samayoga. At the end of this chapter Patanjali mentions that these Siddhis or Fruits are obstacles for Yogis seeking for absolute liberation known as Kaivalya.

Kaivalya Pada (Liberation)

Kaivalya Pada details about the Highest or purest form of mind or chitta and then how many minds manifest from the highest mind due to our ego and Asmita or I-ness. It further describes how a Yogi can attain freedom from the three primary qualities (three Gunas), cause or seed force in our subtle impressions and Karma. Through this process all these three gunas and manifested minds will merge or absorb back into their source from where they have originated. Thus the Yogi attains absolute liberation or Kaivalya.

The Sanskrit Alphabet

The main alphabet used by Sanskrit is known as the Devanāgarī, which can be seen in different ways due to the diverse approaches of different Scholars. Sanskrita is a phonetic language and hence many of us use letters in various orders when we write as we hear from others. Here are the alphabets I have used in this translation.

Sanskrit

Alphabet with English Transliteration

अ	आ	इ	ई	उ	ऊ	
a	ā	i	ī	u	ū	
		ए	ऐ	ओ	औ	
		e	ai	o	au	
ऋ	ॠ	ऌ		अं		अः
ṛ	ṝ	ḷ		aṅ/añ/an/aṃ		aḥ
क	ख	ग	घ	ङ		
ka	kha	ga	gha	ṅa		Guttural
च	छ	ज	झ	ञ		
ca	cha	ja	jha	ña		Palatal
ट	ठ	ड	ढ	ण		
ṭa	ṭha	ḍa	ḍha	ṇa		Cerebral
त	थ	द	ध	न		
ta	tha	da	dha	na		Dental
प	फ	ब	भ	म		
pa	pha	ba	bha	ma		Labial
य	र	ल	व			
ya	ra	la	va			
श	ष	स	ह		क्ष	ज्ञ
śa	ṣa	sa	ha		kṣa	jña

Chapter :1 Samādhi Pāda

अथ योगानुशासनम् ॥१॥

Atha yoga-anushāsanam||1||

Here now begins (atha) the instructions of discipline (anushāsanam) of Yoga (yoga)||1||

This sutra explains Yoga as a path of discipline, also it can be seen as the teachings of yoga beginning once we have mastered some level of discipline in our life.

योगश्चित्तवृत्तिनिरोधः ॥२॥

Yogah-chitta-vṛatti-nirodhaḥ||2||

Yoga (yogaḥ) is the state of cessation or stillness (nirodhaḥ) of the whirlpools (vṛatti) of mind (chitta)||2||

Yoga is stillness or complete cessation of whirlpools of our mind. In the first verse Patanjali mentions Yoga as a Path, while here he mentions Yoga as a goal.

तदा द्रष्टुः स्वरूपेऽवस्थानम् ॥३॥

Tadā draṣṭuḥ svarūpe-avasthānam||3||

Then (tadā), seeker attains state or the oneness (avasthānam) in the essential nature (sva-rūpe) of the Seer (draṣṭuḥ)||3||

Once our mental whirlpools are quietened and we establish our union or awareness of True-Nature (atma-jnana)

वृत्तिसारूप्यमितरत्र ॥४॥

Vṛatti-sārūpyam-itaratra||4||

Otherwise (when we are not in union with our true-self) (itaratra), we identify ourselves or associate with (sārūpyam) the modifications or whirlpools of mind (vṛatti)||4||

If Yoga or Union is highest goal then identifying problems or issues will be the first step towards our goal. It is important to remember that our journey has to begin from where we are. Here Patanjali mentions that we identify ourselves with whirlpools of the mind and their modifications.

वृत्तयः पञ्चतय्यः क्लिष्टा अक्लिष्टाः ॥५॥
Vṛattayaḥ pancha-tayyaḥ kliṣṭā akliṣṭāḥ||5||

The modifications of the mind (vṛttayaḥ), are of 5 types (pañcatayyaḥ), which may be coloured and manipulated, or uncoloured and pure (kliṣṭāḥ akliṣṭāḥ)||5||

Modifications or types of mind-field are five, which can be manipulated or coloured by our past experiences, ego, and i-ness or they can be pure. So fields of the mind can be negative or positive.

प्रमाणविपर्ययविकल्पनिद्रास्मृतयः ॥६॥
Pramāṇa-viparyaya-vikalpa-nidrā-smṛatayaḥ||6||

Direct or valid knowledge or cognition (pramāṇa), false knowledge (viparyaya), imagination or knowledge that is not real (vikalpa), sleep (nidrā) and recollection of past experiences or memory --smṛati-- (smṛatayaḥ) *are the five modifications of mind* ||6||

Five modifications of the mind are valid knowledge, false knowledge, imagination, sleep or lack of awareness, and memory.

प्रत्यक्षानुमानागमाः प्रमाणानि ॥७॥

Pratyakṣā-anumāna-āgamāḥ pramāṇāni||7||

Direct experience (pratyakṣa), assumptions (anumāna) and scriptures or valid sources --āgama-- (āgamāḥ) are the valid or right knowledge (pramāṇāni)||7||

Pramana is the valid or right knowledge we acquire through our direct experience, from assuming and then testifying and from scriptures or valid sources.

विपर्ययो मिथ्याज्ञानमतद्रूपप्रतिष्ठम् ॥८॥

Viparyayo mithyā-jñānam-atad-rūpa-pratiṣṭham||8||

Viparyaya (viparyayaḥ) is wrong knowledge (jñānam) which is not true (mithyā) and this knowledge is based (pratiṣṭham) on mistaking a particular identity for something completely different (atad-rūpa)||8||

Wrong knowledge or Viparyaya is knowing something with false identifications or completely different from its true identity. A typical example is mistakenly seeing a snake in a rope when it is little dark. In Yogic perception identifying our True Self with our physical body or mind is also Viparyaya.

शब्दज्ञानानुपाती वस्तुशून्यो विकल्पः ॥९॥
Śabda-jñāna-anupātī vastu-śūnyo vikalpaḥ||9||

Vikalpa (vikalpaḥ) arises (anupātī) from a verbal (śabda) cognition (jñāna) about something which does not exist or have reality (vastu- śūnyaḥ)||9||

Vikalpa is pure imagination where there are words and thoughts but in reality there is no-object or true existence of them.

अभावप्रत्ययालम्बना वृत्तिर्निद्रा ॥१०॥
Abhāva-pratyaya-ālambanā vṛittir-nidrā||10||

The modification (vṛittiḥ) *known as* Nidrā *or sleep* (nidrā) is based (ālambanā) upon the mental state (pratyaya) of lack (abhāva) of awareness or cognition ||10||

This is state of deep sleep where we have minimum awareness of ourselves and surroundings events.

अनुभूतविषयासम्प्रमोषः स्मृतिः ॥११॥
Anubhūta-viṣayā-asampramoṣaḥ smṛatiḥ||11||

Smṛatiḥ is the recollection of past memories, free from any other sources or vrittis (asampramoṣaḥ), of the objects and subjects (viṣaya) that was *previously* experienced (anubhūta)||11||

Memory is the fifth modification of the mind, which is based on remembering previous experiences.

अभ्यासवैराग्याभ्यां तन्निरोधः ॥१२॥
Abhyāsa-vairājna-abhyāṁ tan-nirodhaḥ||12||

Through dedicated practice (abhyāsa) and detachment or renunciation (vairājna) one can attain stillness or cessation (nirodhaḥ) of the five modifications of the mind. ||12||

Here Patanjali gives us tools or remedies to deal with mental modifications. These are Abhyasa meaning sincere practice and Vairajna meaning detachment from all the worldly associations and pleasure seeking desires in material objects.

तत्र स्थितौ यत्नोऽभ्यासः॥१३॥
Tatra sthitau yatno'-abhyāsaḥ||13||

Abhyāsa or practice (abhyāsaḥ) is the effort (yatnaḥ) to attain to that (tatra) state (sthiti) of mental peace (sthitau)||13||

Abhyasa or Practice of Ashtanga Yoga or Raja Yoga practices will lead us to a state of a peaceful or focussed mind free from modifications or whirlpools.

स तु दीर्घकालनैरन्तर्यसत्कारासेवितो दृढभूमिः॥१४॥
Sa tu dīrgha-kāla-nairantarya-satkāra-asevito dṛḍha-bhūmiḥ||14||

When that *practice* (saḥ), sincerely followed or practised (sevitaḥ) regularly without interruption (nairantarya) and true (sat) dedicated attitude (kārā) for a long (dīrgha) time (kāla), will certainly (tu) attain firm (dṛḍha) foundation or success (bhūmiḥ) in Yoga ||14||

Swamiji Dr Gitananda Giriji says that success in yoga can be achieved through dedicated sadhana with REGULARITY, REPETITION, AND RHYTHM.

दृष्टानुश्रविकविषयवितृष्णस्य वशीकारसञ्ज्ञा वैराग्यम् ॥१५॥

Dṛaṣṭā-anuśravika-viṣaya-vitṛaṣṇasya vaśīkāra-sañjñā vairājnam||15||

Detachment or Renunciation (vairāgyam) is known (sañjñā) as to be free from (vaśīkāra) the desires (vitṛṣṇasya) for objects or material (viṣaya) seen or known(dṛaṣṭa) or repeatedly heard or described in the scriptures (ānuśravika)||15||
Detachment is to free ourselves from all the desires, ego and i-ness seeking pleasure or fulfilment from objects, or material possessions.

तत्परं पुरुषख्यातेर्गुणवैतृष्ण्यम् ॥१६॥

Tatparaṁ puruṣha-khyāter-guṇa-vaitṛṣṇyam||16||

Freeing our mind (vaitṛaṣṇyam) from actions or responses driven by the Guṇa-s, *(the three primary qualities of nature)* (guṇa), through knowledge (khyāteḥ) of Self or Soul (puruṣa) is known as the highest detachment or *Vairājna* (tad param)||16||

As Lord Krishna explains in Bhagavat Gita .... all our actions, choices and mental activities are driven from the three primary qualities of nature (sattva-purity, or light, rajas-action, and tamas- inertia or darkness). Knowing that all the materials objects and impermanent and knowing the eternal souls or Purusha is the highest form of Vairajna.

वितर्कविचारानन्दास्मितारूपानुगमात्सम्प्रज्ञातः ॥१७॥
Vitarka-vichāra-ānanda-asmitā-rūpa-anugamāt-samprajñātaḥ||17||

Samādhi or state of awareness with self-identification (samprajñātaḥ) *can be achieved* through (anugamāt) practices of reasoning (Vitarka), contemplations and discrimination (Vichāra), Joyfulness (Ānanda) and awareness of I-ness (Asmitā) ||17||

This is the first category level of Samadhi or higher conscious experience. In this Samadhi there is still the identity of 'I' and the sense is there and can be achieved through reasoning, discrimination, joyfulness and awareness of I-ness.

विरामप्रत्ययाभ्यासपूर्वः संस्कारशेषोऽन्यः ॥१८॥
Virāma-pratyaya-abhyāsa-pūrvaḥ saṁskāra-śeṣounyaḥ||18||
The second type of Samādhi (anyaḥ) can be attained (pūrvaḥ) by the practice (abhyāsa) of stilling or quietening (virāma) the mental fluctuations (pratyaya), *which is the natural fruit of mastering the Vairājna, but the latent impressions* (saṁskāra) *are still there* (śeṣaḥ) this is known as Asamprajnata samadhi ||18||

This is a further advanced state of Samadhi or Self-Realisation where Sadhaka becomes free from attachment with all the mundane associations, but there are still some subtle impressions of habitual seeds of thoughts and desires.

भवप्रत्ययो विदेहप्रकृतिलयानाम् ॥१९॥
Bhava-pratyayo Videha-prakṛati-layānām||19||

Some who have attained higher levels of Samadhi (Videha- free from body or object) or who have experienced and known True or Real Nature (prakṛtilayānām) will be born again in this world ......? if there are any subtle impressions or Samaskaras (bhava) *or ignorance is remaining.* ||19||

Even when we have attained Samprajnata or Asamprajnata Samadhi, Patanjali says that as long as there are any subtle impressions of chitta-vrittis or ignorance .... remaining, under the influence of primary nature or qualities, we are bound to be born again.

श्रद्धावीर्यस्मृतिसमाधिप्रज्ञापूर्वक इतरेषाम् ॥२०॥
Śraddhā-vīrya-smṛati-samādhi-prajñā-pūrvaka itareṣām||20||

One who follows the path .... using Yoga Kriyas and Prakriyas or methods (Upayas) (itareṣām), *with conscious effort is followed with* (pūrvakaḥ) faith (śraddhā), zeal and will (vīrya), recollection and remembering (smṛati), highest union or self-realisation (samādhi). True knowledge or wisdom (prajñā) will be attained ||20||

Faith in practice, directing positive energy and zeal in the path, repeated memory or contemplation of the path and processes or practices, training in the deepest levels of meditation, acquiring and realising Truth or Real nature or knowledge is the?? five fold path for others to achieve samadhi or union.

तीव्रसंवेगानामासन्नः ॥२१॥

Tīvra-saṁvegānām-āsannaḥ||21||

This Samadhi, by practising the above, can be attained (āsannaḥ) *by people more quickly through the* intense (tīvra) desire for spiritual evolution (saṁvegānām)||21||

Those who pursue their practices with intensity, momentum and enthusiasm will achieve samadhi or the fruits thereof more quickly, compared to those of medium or lesser intensity.

मृदुमध्याधिमात्रत्वात्ततोऽपि विशेषः ॥२२॥

Mṛadu-madhya-adhimātratvāt-tato-api visheṣaḥ||22||

Intensity of Sadhana or practice because of approach which can be easy, or gentle (mṛadu), moderate or medium (madhya) and intense or advanced dedicated or speedy (adhimātratvāt), which consequently .... (tatas) in differences make it special (viśeṣaḥ) *(among those sadhakas seeking...... spiritual realisations)* (api)||22||

This verse explains three subdivisions of practice or sadhana, which is of mild intensity, medium intensity, and intense intensity.

ईश्वरप्रणिधानाद्वा ॥२३॥

Īśvara-praṇidhānād-vā||23||

Otherwise (vā) *one can attain Samadhi* through profound faith, devotion and dedication (praṇidhānāt) to Divine or Higher Consciousness (īśvara)||23||

With devotion, contemplation and surrendering or letting go into the creative source from which we emerge, attaining samadhi is imminent. Swamiji Dr Gitananda Giri Ji translates this by using the term- Īśvara-prashādana which means seeing the life as divine blessings and dedicating it to divine cause.

क्लेशकर्मविपाकाशयैरपरामृष्टः पुरुषविशेष ईश्वरः ॥२४॥

Kleśha-karma-vipākā-śayaira-parāmṛaṣṭaḥ purusha-viśeṣa īśvaraḥ||24||

Īśvara (īśvaraḥ) is a particular and special (viśeṣaḥ) divine consciousness (puruṣha) which is unaffected (aparāmṛṣṭaḥ) by whirlpools or modifications of the mind and afflictions-- (klesha), all the actions (karma), the fruits of actions (vipāka) or the resulting latent subtle impressions or samaskaras (āśayaiḥ)||24||

That divine or creative source is higher consciousness, that is unaffected by colourings (kleshas), actions (karmas), or results of those actions that happen when latent impressions stir and cause those actions.

तत्र निरतिशयं सर्वज्ञवीजम्॥२५॥

Tatra niratiśayaṁ sarvajña-vījam||25||

In that or there (tatra), the Omniscient, all knowing (sarvajña) Seed (vījam) cannot be exceeded, surpassed or grow any further (niratiśayam)||25||

As the Isvara or divine conscious is subtlest and purest and all that manifest from this cannot exceed any higher than this.

पूर्वेषामपि गुरुः कालेनानवच्छेदात्॥२६॥

Pūrveṣām-api guruḥ kālenān-avacchedāt||26||

That divine consciousness is the Guru (guruḥ- one who leads from darkness to light) even (api) of the well-known masters (pūrveṣām), because that divine is undetermined or unlimited (anavacchedāt) by Time (kālena)||26||

Lord Krishna in Bhagavat Gita says that consciousness is eternal and nothing can effect it, like fire cannot burn it, water cannot wet it, air cannot dry it, sword cannot cut it. Here Patanjali says that Divine Consciousness is Highest Guru of even all the masters and it is beyond time, cause, and limitations.

तस्य वाचकः प्रणवः॥२७॥

Tasya vāchakaḥ praṇavaḥ||27||

Pranava AUM (praṇavaḥ) is the verbal or sound (vācakaḥ) of that (tasya) divine consciousness ||27||

Pranava AUM or OM is the sacred sound or vibration representing this divine or creative source- Isvara.

तज्जपस्तदर्थभावनम्॥२८॥

Tajjapas-tada-artha-bhāvanam||28||

Pranava Sadhana for Samadhi can be followed by the repetitive chanting (japaḥ) of that *OM* (tad) the meditation or contemplation (bhāvanam) on its (tad) meaning (artha)||28||

To attain Samadhi through Pranava sadhana, one must chant the mantra AUM with focussing the mind on its meaning or essence experiencing the divinity in vibration.

ततः प्रत्यक्चेतनाधिगमोऽप्यन्तरायाभावश्च॥२९॥

Tataḥ pratyak-chetanā-adhigamah-api-antarāya-abhāvash-cha||29||

From the above Sadhana of Pranava (tatas) *we attain the* realization (adhigamaḥ) of one›s own Real Self (pratyak-chetana) as well as (api... cha) the removal (abhāvaḥ) of obstacles (antarāya)||29||

Pranava Sadhana fruits in Self-realisation as well as it also helps removing the obstacles holding us away from our spiritual evolution.

व्याधिस्त्यानसंशयप्रमादालस्याविरतिभ्रान्तिदर्शनालब्ध
भूमिकत्वानवस्थितत्वानि चित्तविक्षेपास्तेऽन्तरायाः॥३०॥
Vyādhi-styāna-saṁshaya-pramāda-alasya-avirati-
bhrānti-darshan-alabdha-bhūmikatva-anavasthi-tatvāni
chitta-vikṣepās-te-antarāyāḥ||30||

Disease (vyādhi), lack of mental interest or dullness (styāna), doubt (saṁshaya), negligence (pramāda), laziness (ālasya), lack of control of sensual desires (avirati), wrong knowledge or perception (bhrānti-darshana), inability to attain or achieve to any Yogic experiences or states (alabdha-bhūmikatva) and unsteadiness or lack of stability- (anavasthi-tatvāni) are those (te) nine the obstacles (antarāyāḥ) of mental calmness or stillness (citta-vikṣepāḥ) ||30||

Nine types of obstacles destructing - (do you mean destroying or deconstructing?) or deviating our mind from the yoga path are physical illness, idleness or procrastination, doubt or lack of faith, carelessness, laziness or lethargy, material desires or cravings, false views or perceptions, failing to attain or recognise stages of the practice or progress, and inability to maintain states already achieved.

दुःखदौर्मनस्याङ्गमेजयत्वश्वासप्रश्वासा
विक्षेपसहभुवः ॥३१॥
Duḥkha-daurmanasya-aṅga-mejayatva-shvāsa-prashvāsā
vikṣepa-sahabhuvaḥ||31||

Pain (duḥkha), misery (daurmanasya), shakiness or trembling of body limbs (aṅgam-ejayatva), disturbed or laboured breathing (śvāsa-praśvāsāḥ,) appear or arise (bhuvaḥ) together (saha) as the result of disturbances (vikṣepa) due to obstacles ||31||

Pain, discomfort, miserable feelings, restless or trembling of limbs and disturbed breathing are all together outcomes of obstacles in our life and sadhana.

तत्प्रतिषेधार्थमेकतत्त्वाभ्यासः ॥३२॥
Tat-pratiṣedha-artham-eka-tattva-abhyāsaḥ||32||

For the goal of (artham) keeping away from obstacles or to overcome them (tad-pratiṣedha), the dedicated practice or sadhana (abhyāsaḥ) of single-pointed focus (eka) one principle (tattva) *should be followed* ||32||

To overcome or avoid obstacles one must to follow single-pointedness or focus on one principle or path which are described in following Sutras.

मैत्रीकरुणामुदितोपेक्षाणां सुखदुःखपुण्यापुण्यविषयाणां भावनातश्चित्तप्रसादनम् ॥३३॥

Maitrī-karuṇā-mudita-upekṣāṇāṁ sukha-duḥkha-puṇya-apuṇya-viṣayāṇāṁ bhāvanātah-chitta-prasādanam||33||

Peace of mind is fruit (chitta-prasādanam) of contemplation and followings (bhāvanātaḥ) of friendliness (maitrī), compassion (karuṇā), joyfulness (muditā) and indifference or equanimity (upekṣāṇām) regarding or in contexts (viṣayāṇām) *pleasure or likings* (sukha), suffering, distress or disliking (duḥkha), pure (puṇya) *and* impure (apuṇya) *respectively*||33||

The mind becomes purified or free from obstacles by cultivating and practicing friendliness towards those who are happy, compassion for those who are suffering, goodwill towards those who are virtuous, and equanimity or neutrality towards those we perceive as wicked or evil.

प्रच्छर्दनविधारणाभ्यां वा प्राणस्य ॥३४॥

Pracchardana-vidhāraṇābhyāṁ vā prāṇasya||34||

Or (vā) *this peace of mind can be attained* by refining or controlling flow (pracchardana) and retention (vidhāraṇābhyām) of Prāṇa, the vital universal energy (prāṇasya)||34||

The one-pointedness is also achieved by regulating the breath to refine, control and retain Prana. Prana is the subtlest, eternal all-pervading vital universal force.

विषयवती वा प्रवृत्तिरुत्पन्ना मनसः स्थितिनिबन्धिनी ॥३५॥

Vishayavatī vā pravṛatti-rutpannā manasaḥ sthiti-nibandhinī||35||

Or (vā) that single-pointedness can be attained through a higher perception (pravṛattiḥ) relating to subjects and objects of experiences (viṣayavatī), at the moment when it emerges (utpannā) which brings (nibandhinī) state (sthiti) of calmness of mind (manasaḥ) ||35||

Witnessing the mind on sensory experiences (senses and mind) or perceptions when they arise or take place and focussing the mind on inner higher perceptions and reality will also lead to one-pointed and tranquil mind.

विशोका वा ज्योतिष्मती ॥३६॥

Vishokā vā jyotiṣmatī||36||

Or (vā) *this peace of mind can also be attained through perceiving the* luminous light (jyotiṣmatī) which is free from sorrow (viśokā) ||36||

We can also attain single-pointedness or peace of mind by focussing the mind on inner light or effulgence, or luminosity free from sufferings.

वीतरागविषयं वा चित्तम् ॥३७॥

Vītarāga-viṣayaṁ vā chittam||37||

Or (vā) *focussing* the mind (chittam) on subjects, thought, or teachings (viṣayam) of masters or Yogi's freeing us from a sage passions and desires for material objects (vītarāga) *can also bring single-pointedness or peace of mind* ||37||

Contemplating or meditating on subjects, concepts and great Yogi's and masters freeing us from desires and attachment also leads us to a single-pointed mind.

स्वप्ननिद्राज्ञानालम्बनं वा ॥३८॥

Svapna-nidrā-jñāna-alambanaṁ vā||38||

Or (vā) taking support (ālambanam) of the knowledges in forms of words, shapes and qualities (jñāna) *experienced* in dreams (svapna) or in the state of deep sleep (nidrā) *can also lead us to peace of mind and single-pointedness* ||38||

Also by focusing on the dreams and sleep states and their nature, the mind becomes stabilised and tranquil.

यथाभिमतध्यानाद्वा ॥३९॥

Yathā-abhimata-dhyānādvā||39||

Or (vā) by meditating (dhyānāt) on a suitable yogic practice or principle that one likes (yathā-abhimata) one can attain single-pointedness of mind ||39||

Contemplating or concentrating our mind on one yogic practice or principle, which you can choose according to your ability and suitability one can attain a stable and tranquil mind.

परमाणुपरममहत्त्वान्तोऽस्य वशीकारः ॥४०॥

Paramāṇu-parama-mahattva-anto-asya vashīkāraḥ||40||

When gone through the above practices the mind attains ability to focus on subtlest of elements (paramāṇu) as well as up to (antaḥ) infinitely or largest that exist (parama-mahattva), then Sadhaka attains complete mastery (vaśīkāraḥ) over it or mind (asya) ||40||

Here Patanjali explains the fruits of single-pointed awareness. Through such practices (described in 1.33-1.39), the mind develops the power of becoming aware or experiences of the smallest size object (atom) as well as on the largest (the whole universe itself), achieves mastery or awareness of subtlest and largest particles. This is complete mastery of our mind.

क्षीणवृत्तेरभिजातस्येव मणेर्ग्रहीतृग्रहणग्राह्येषु तत्स्थतदञ्जनता समापत्तिः॥४१॥

Kṣīṇa-vṛatter-abhijātasya-va maṇeh-grahītṛa-grahaṇa-grāhyeṣu tat-stha-tad-añjanatā samāpattiḥ||41||

When fluctuations (vratteh) are refined or quietened (kṣīṇa) then gradually stability of mind (abhijātasya), *this is* like (iva) clarity or transparency in awareness of the mind (maṇeḥ) in respect to the knower (grahītṛa), the instruments of knowledge (grahaṇa) and what is to be known (grāhyeṣu) which are all objects of mental awareness. This state of awareness of reality (tad-stha-tad-añjanatā) is known as Samāpatti (samāpattiḥ)||41||

When the modifications of the mind have become weakened, the mind becomes like a transparent clear awareness, and thus can easily experience the qualities of whatever object is being observed, as well as the mind being able to distinguish between the observer, the means of observing, and what is to be the object observed. This state of Samadhi, Union or awareness is known as samapattih.

शब्दार्थज्ञानविकल्पैः सङ्कीर्णा सवितर्का समापत्तिः ॥४२॥

Śabda-artha-jñāna-vikalpaiḥ saṅkīrṇā savitarkā samāpattiḥ||42||

Thoughtful Samadhi or awareness is (savitarkā samāpattiḥ) is that which is combined (saṅkīrṇā) of ideas, options or thoughts (vikalpaiḥ) of between word (śabda), *it's* meaning (artha) and the knowledge (jñāna)||42||

One type of such union (samapattih) is one with thoughtfulness in which there is a mixture of three things, a word or name going with the object, the meaning or identity of that object, and the knowledge associated with that object; this union is known as savitarka samapattih.

स्मृतिपरिशुद्धौ स्वरूपशून्येवार्थमात्रनिर्भासा निर्वितर्का ॥४३॥

Smṛati-pariśuddhau svarūpa-shūnyeva-artha-mātra-nirbhāsā nirvitarkā||43||

When memory (smṛti) is absolutely purified (pariśuddhau), as it becomes (iva), devoid of free from (śūnyā) of its own essential nature (sva-rūpa), *that Samādhi* in which only (mātra) the object or awareness (artha) shines forth (nirbhāsā) is known as Nirvitarkā (nirvitarkā)||43||

When the memory or mental impressions are purified, then the mind becomes free from its own nature and only the object on which it is contemplating appears to shine forward; this type of union is known as nirvitarka samapattih or thoughtless-awareness.

एतयैव सविचारा निर्विचारा च सूक्ष्मविषया व्याख्याता ॥४४॥

Etayā-eva savichārā nirvichārā ca sūkṣma-viṣayā vyākhyātā||44||

By means these previous explanation (etayā) *(the Samādhi is known as thoughtful* (savichārā) and (ca) free from thoughts or mental impressions (nirvichārā), whose objects or subjects (viṣayā) are subtle (sūkṣma), are also (eva) explained (vyākhyātā)||44||

The Samadhi with subtle objects is known as savichara and nirvichara samapattih and also operates in the same way as it operates with gross objects in savitarka samapattih.

सूक्ष्मविषयत्वं चालिङ्गपर्यवसानम् ॥४५॥

Sūkṣma-viṣaya-tvaṁ cha-aliṅga-paryavasānam||45||

And (cha) being the subtle in quality (sūkṣma) in regards to object (viṣayatvam) *in comparison to previous once one attains* ends (paryavasānam) the union or awareness of the Un-manifested (true potentials) Prakṛati (aliṅga)||45||

Attaining such union or Samadhi with subtle objects extends all the way up to awareness of realisation of un-manifested prakriti or potentials of the subtlest elements.

ता एव सवीजः समाधिः।।४६।।

Tā eva sabījaḥ samādhiḥ||46||

Only (eva) those (tāḥ) (four above described types of Samadhis -*Savitarkā, Nirvitarkā, Savichārā and Nirvichārā) are also known as Samadhi with seed or object of awareness* (sabījaḥ samādhiḥ) ||46||

These four types of samadhis are the only kinds of unions or realisations (samadhi) which are objective, and have a seed of an object.

निर्विचारवैशारद्येऽध्यात्मप्रसादः।।४७।।

Nirvichāra-vaishāradye-adhyātma-prasādaḥ||47||

On mastering skills or proficiency (vaiśāradye) in Nirvichāra Samādhi (nirvichāra), it brings the purity (prasādaḥ) in the inner instruments of awareness (Manas or mind and Buddhi or Intellect) which fruits in Spiritual realisations (adhyātma) ||47||

As one gains proficiency in the undisturbed flow in nirvichara, a purity and luminosity of the inner instrument of mind is attained. This is spiritual fruit of above Samadhis.

ऋतम्भरा तत्र प्रज्ञा ॥४८॥
Ṛitambharā tatra prajñā||48||

The True knowledge or wisdom (prajñā) *attained* in that *(Nirvichāra samādhi or Nirvichārā Samāpatti)* (tatra) *is known as* Ṛitambharā (ṛitambharā)||48||

The experience that is attained in that state is full of wisdom and of Truth and Reality.

श्रुतानुमानप्रज्ञाभ्यामन्यविषया विशेषार्थत्वात् ॥४९॥
Śruta-anumāna-prajñā-abhyām-anya-viṣayā visheṣa-arthatvāt||49||

That Prajñā or highest knowledge gained is different (anyaviṣayā) from knowledges (prajñābhyām) attained through listening (śruta) or inference (anumāna), because it is particularly from true experience of characteristics (viśeṣa) of objects and their qualities (arthatvāt)||49||

That highest form of knowledge is different from the knowledge that is acquired with testimony or through inference, because it relates directly to the specifics of the object, rather than to those words or other concepts. This verse explains that your own experience is far more special and valuable then knowing from outer sources.

तज्जः संस्कारोऽन्यसंस्कारप्रतिबन्धी ॥५०॥

Tajjaḥ saṁskārah-anyas-aṁskāra-pratibandhī||50||

The latent impression (saṁskāraḥ) born (jaḥ) of that *Prajñā arisen in Nirvichāra samādhi* (tad) obstructs or removes (pratibandhī) the other (anya) latent impressions (saṁskāra)||50||

This type of knowledge of reality and truth also creates latent impressions in the mind-field, but these new positive spiritual impressions tend to remove, reduce or obstruct the formation of other less useful forms of habitual latent impressions.

तस्यापि निरोधे सर्वनिरोधान्निर्वीजः समाधिः ॥५१॥

Tasya-api nirodhe sarva-nirodhān-nirbījaḥ samādhiḥ||51||

On the cessation (nirodhe) of those latent impressions arising from Praja or higher wisdom (tasya) too (api), there is highest form of Samadhi , where awareness of true-self becomes free from awareness of object of focus too is known as (nirbījaḥ samādhiḥ) through the cessation (nirodhāt) of all *lower and higher mental modifications or fluctuations* (sarva)||51||

When even these latent impressions from the highest Truth and Reality dissolves or cease along with the other impressions, then Sadhaka attains seedless or objectless union or concentration.

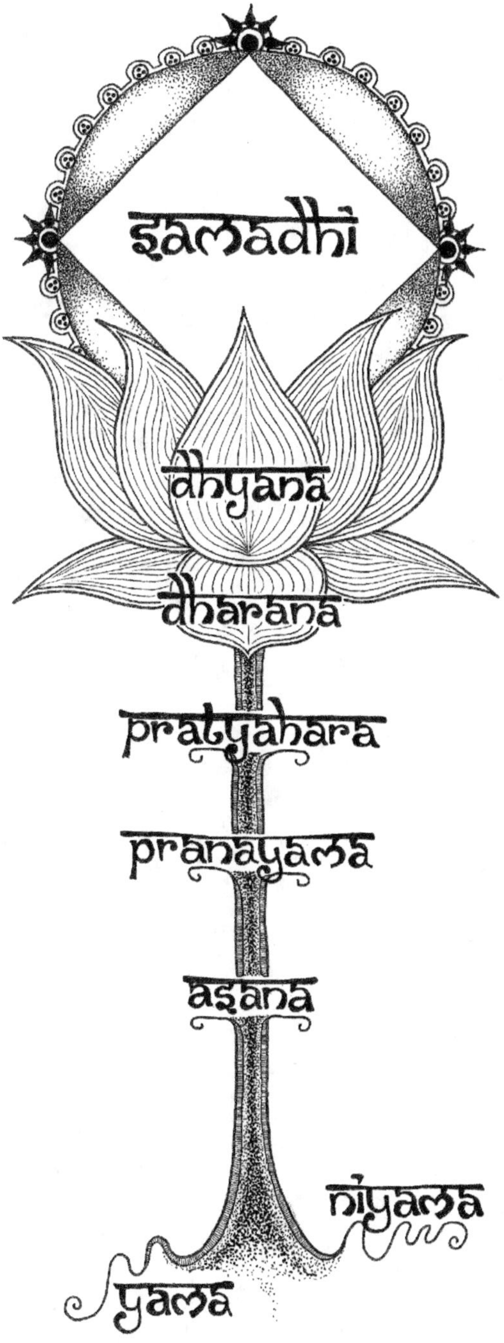
samadhi
dhyana
dharana
pratyahara
pranayama
asana
niyama
yama

Chapter 2: Sādhanā Pāda

तपःस्वाध्यायेश्वरप्रणिधानानि क्रियायोगः॥१॥
Tapaḥ-svādhyāya-iśvara-praṇidhānāni kriya-yogaḥ||1||

Austerity, Penance or dedicated sadhana (tapas), Introspection, self-awareness and study of scriptures (svādhyāya) *and* Devotion, faith and dedicated all our actions to divine cause (īśvara-praṇidhānāni) together are known as Kriyā yoga or Yoga of Action (kriya-yogaḥ)||1||

Yoga in the form of action (kriya yoga) has three elements to follow: 1) practice and austerity (tapas), 2) self-study and self-reflection in respect of practices (svadhyaya), and 3) devotion and offering or dedicating all our actions to the creative divine consciousness from which we manifested (ishvara pranidhana).

समाधिभावनार्थः क्लेशतनूकरणार्थश्च॥२॥
Samādhi-bhāvana-arthaḥ klesha-tanū-karaṇa-arthash cha||2||

Aim of Kriya Yoga (arthaḥ... arthaḥ) is to attain or experience (bhāvana) Samādhi or Union (samādhi) and (ca) removing or purifying (tanū-karaṇa) the Kleshas (kleśa)||2||

That Kriya Yoga should be practiced to reach samadhi and minimize the mental impressions and thought patterns (kleshas).

अविद्यास्मितारागद्वेषाभिनिवेशाः पञ्च क्लेशाः ॥३॥
Avidyā-asmitā-rāga-dveṣa-abhiniveśāḥ pañcha kleshāḥ||3||

Ignorance *or lack of True Knowledge* (avidyā), egoism or I-ness (asmitā), attraction for pleasure seeking objects (rāga), aversion from practices or things need to be done (dveṣa) and fear of death or clinging on to things that need to be let go (abhiniveshāḥ) are the five (pañcha) Kleshas or Afflictions or impure mental impressions (kleshāḥ)||3||

There are five kinds of mental impressions or afflictions (kleshas): 1) ignorance- not knowing the truth or ignoring the truth we know (avidya), 2) I-ness, individuality, or egoism (asmita), 3) attachment or addiction to mental impressions or objects (raga), 4) aversion to thought patterns or objects (dvesha), and 5) clinging to life or objects at any cost as well as fear of loss or death.

अविद्या क्षेत्रमुत्तरेषां प्रसुप्ततनुविच्छिन्नोदाराणाम् ॥४॥
Avidyā kṣetram-uttareṣāṁ prasupta-tanu-vicchinna-
udārāṇām||4||

Ignorance (avidyā) is the cause force
or field (kṣetram) for the other *four
Kleshas* (uttareṣām) *and they can be*
dormant (prasupta), subtle and sub-conscious (tanu),
interrupted or occasional (vicchinna) or active and
affective (udārāṇām)||4||

Ignorance is the root cause for the other four kleshas or afflictions and each one of them have four states or levels- : 1) dormant or inactive, 2) weak, or subconscious 3) interrupted or in gaps, or 4) active and producing afflicted thoughts or actions to varying degrees.

अनित्याशुचिदुःखानात्मसु नित्यशुचिसुखात्मख्यातिरविद्
या॥५॥

Anita-ashuchi-duḥkha-anātmasu nitya-shuchi-sukha-atma-khyātira-vidyā||5||

Ignorance (avidyā) is to consider or seeing (khyātiḥ) the Truth or Reality and permanence (nitya) what is subject to change (anitya), and also seeing as pure (shuchi) in what is not pure (ashuchi), or seeking pleasure (sukha) in what is unpleasant or painful (duḥkha) and knowing the Self (ātma) in what is the not the Self (anātmasu)||5||

Ignorance (avidya) is : 1) seeing or perceiving non-eternal as eternal, 2) mistaking the impure for pure, 3) mistaking something to bring happiness which brings misery, and 4) knowing unreal to be real or self. Avidya is our manipulated perception or knowledge of True Self (atman) and what is good and what is not good for our evolution. Swamiji Dr Gitananda Giri Ji mentions that "what is good for you may not be always pleasant, and what is pleasant may be not be good for you. Make sure we never avoid good for sake of pleasure."

Swamiji Dr Gitanand Giriji also says that "for a yogi ignorance is not only lack of knowledge but also denying the truth we know."

दृग्दर्शनशक्त्योरेकात्मतेवास्मिता ॥६॥

Dṛig-darshana-shaktyor-ekātmata-iva-asmitā||6||

Egoism or I-ness (asmitā) is affliction or manipulation (iva) of the identification or knowledge (ekātmatā) of the cognition or experience (dṛig) under the influence or power (shaktyoḥ) with the view-points (darshana) under power(shaktyoḥ) from Individual Intellect, ego or self-pleasing principles ||6||

The klesha of I-ness or egoism (asmita) arises from ignorance, occurs due to the mistake of taking the intellect (buddhi, which knows, decides, judges, and discriminates) as the pure consciousness (purusha/drig). Asmita or egoism is perceiving or seeing things according to our own ego our limited mind and not the way the are in their own true nature.

सुखानुशयी रागः ॥७॥

Sukhānuśayī rāgaḥ||7||

Attachment (rāgaḥ) is that which results (anuśayī) from pleasure seeking objects (sukha) ||7||

Raga is attraction or attachment for objects and activities bringing pleasure to our senses and mind.

दुःखानुशयी द्वेषः॥८॥
Duḥkha-anushayī dveṣaḥ||8||

Aversion (dveṣaḥ) is the result or outcome (anushayī) from pain, sorrow or that which we don't like (duḥkha) ||8||

This aversion or repulsion keeps us away from many good things, virtues and practices we need to follow, as in the beginning they might not seem very pleasant.

स्वरसवाही विदुषोऽपि तथारूढोऽभिनिवेशः॥९॥
Svarasavāhī viduṣo-api tathā-ārūḍho-abhiniveshaḥ||9||

The inborn or inherited with birth (svarasavāhī) fear of death or losing what we possess (abhiniveshaḥ) is established or deeply rooted (ārūḍhaḥ) in like an essential manner (tathā), even (api) in the wise or realised one (viduṣaḥ)||9||

Even for those people who are learned or mastered, there is an ever-lasting, and firm clinging or fear of letting go of material and non-material aspects of life at any cost seems to be part of existence.

ते प्रतिप्रसवहेयाः सूक्ष्माः ॥१०॥

Te pratiprasava-heyāḥ sūkṣamāḥ||10||

Those (te) subtle *Kleshas or afflictions* (sūkṣmāḥ) are to be removed or let go (heyāḥ) through cessation of activities of the mind (pratiprasava)||10||

When the five types of modifications (kleshas) are in their subtle, or are in merely potential form, they must be dissolved through letting go from the consciousness itself for complete cessation. These afflictions are easy to remove at the very beginning, like the weeds in your garden to be removed at the very beginning when first sprouting. Once these Kleshas become potential, they take over our Buddhi-intellect and conscious-self.

ध्यानहेयास्तद्वृत्तयः ॥११॥

Dhyāna-heyas-tad-vṛattayaḥ||11||

The *afflictive* modifications of mind (vṛttayaḥ) of those Kleshas afflictions (tad) can be abandoned or removed (heyāḥ) through meditation (dhyāna)||11||

These modifications of the mind at a time when they are afflictive or have some potency of impressions (klishta), they are to be removed and let go through meditation (Dhyana).

क्लेशमूलः कर्माशयो दृष्टादृष्टजन्मवेदनीयः॥१२॥

Klesha-mūlaḥ karma-ashayo dṛaṣṭa-adṛaṣṭa-janma-vedanīyaḥ||12||

Latent impression as outcomes of our actions (karma-āshayaḥ), which rooted (mūlaḥ) from Kleshas or Afflictions (klesha), becomes manifested (vedanīyaḥ) in this life time (dṛaṣṭa-janma) or in a future life time (adṛaṣṭa-janma)||12||

Latent impressions or modifications that are afflicted as a result from other actions (karmas) and were caused by Kleshas, may become active and experienced in a present life time or a future life time at some point.

Lots of our Karmas and Actions are caused by the influence of Kleshas and we accumulate them as Seed Karma. These seed karmas will become active when it's the right opportunity for them. You can understand it by looking at flowers or fruit trees, how they wait for right season and ideal conditions to bring forth flowers and fruits.

सति मूले तद्विपाको जात्यायुर्भोगाः ॥१३॥

Sati mūle tad-vipāko jāti-āyur-bhogāḥ||13||

As long as these Kleshas or Afflictions are remaining (sati) at the root (mūle), the consequences or results (vipākaḥ) of it (tad) are birth (jāti), span of life (āyus) and experiences one has to go through (bhogāḥ)||13||

IF there are even traces of these Kleshas remain at the subtlest level, one has to go through life-birth cycles which brings results in type of birth, span of life and experiences one has to go through. Here Kleshas are seen as the root cause behind our Karma or actions and birth, life span and experiences are outcomes or fruits of actions or Karma.

ते ह्लादपरितापफलाः पुण्यापुण्यहेतुत्वात् ॥१४॥

Te hlāda-paritāpphalāḥ puṇya-apuṇya-hetutvāt||14||

On account or outcomes (hetutvāt) of virtues (puṇya) and non-virtues (apuṇya), those (birth, span of life and experience) (te) the fruits will appear or manifest as (phalāḥ) of pleasure (hlāda) or of pain (paritāpa)||14||

Kleshas and Karmas which are of good virtue will bring pleasant fruits while once which are of no good virtue will bring painful experiences.

परिणामतापसंस्कारदुःखैर्गुणवृत्तिविरोधाच्च दुःखमेव सर्वं विवेकिनः ॥१५॥

Pariṇāma-tāpa-saṁskāra-duḥkhair-guṇa-vṛatti-virodhāch-cha duḥkhameva sarvaṁ vivekinaḥ||15||

For people with ability to discriminate (vivekinaḥ), everything (sarvam) is *considered as* (eva) painful (duḥkham) because of the sufferings (duḥkhaiḥ) resulting as consequences *of one's own actions* (pariṇāma) and painful experiences (tāpa) *and* the deep ingrained latent impressions (saṁskāra), as well as also (ca) from the two opposit (virodhāt) whirlpools of mind (pleasant-painful, like-dislike, attraction-repulsion)(vṛatti) of the dominance of primary qualities (guṇa)||15||

A wise, discriminating person will see all worldly experiences as painful and try to remain in balance or equanimity in every situation, because of reasoning that all these experiences lead to more consequences, anxiety, and deep behaviour patterns or habits (samskaras), as well as acting in opposition to natural qualities.

हेयं दुःखमनागतम् ॥१६॥

Heyaṁ duḥkham-anāgatam||16||

Pain or miseries (duḥkham) yet to come in future (anāgatam) must be avoided (heyam)||16||

By using discriminative reasoning one can avoid miseries or pain yet to come in life. This will help Sadhaka avoid a series of Kleshas and Karmas. I like the phrase for this verse- "always be prepared to prevent, so you don't have to repair and repaint."

द्रष्टृदृश्ययोः संयोगो हेयहेतुः ॥१७॥

Draṣṭṛa-dṛashyayoḥ saṁyogah heya-hetuḥ||17||

The union or attachment (saṁyogaḥ) of the Sadhaka or Seer (draṣṭṛ) with what to be seen or experienced (dṛśyayoḥ) is the cause (hetuḥ) of that which is to be abandoned or avoided (heya)||17||

Here Patanjali mentions that a seeker should be free from any attachment with objects and their experiences.

प्रकाशक्रियास्थितिशीलं भूतेन्द्रियात्मकं भोगापवर्गार्थं दृश्यम् ॥१८॥

Prakāsha-kriyā-sthiti-shīlaṁ bhūta-indriya-ātmakaṁ bhoga-apavarga-arthaṁ dṛashyam||18||

Objects to be known or seen (dṛśyam) is by nature (shīlam) are illuminatory (prakāsha), changeable (kriyā) and have a place (sthiti). *Secondly,* it consists (ātmakam) of elements (which are subtle and gross) (bhūta) *and* have the power of perceiving and actions (Jnanendriyas and Karmendriyas) (indriya). *Lastly it has the aim or means* (artham) of experience (bhoga) and Liberation (apavarga)||18||

The objects to be known or experienced by Sadhaka are by their nature of: 1) illumination or sentience, 2) activity or mutability, and 3) inertia or status; they contain the elements and the powers of the senses, and exist for the purpose of experiencing the world and for liberation or enlightenment. In this Sutra Patanjali explains that Sadhaka should try to be aware of all these objects of experiences like sense organs, mind, intellect and consciousness (atma-jnana)

विशेषाविशेषलिङ्गमात्रालिङ्गानि गुणपर्वाणि ॥१९॥
Visheṣā-visheṣa-liṅga-mātra-aliṅgāni guṇa-parvāṇi||19||

The types or results of various compositions (parvāṇi) of the Guṇas (guṇa) *are specific and different* (visheṣa), similar or non-specific (avisheṣa), subtlest or indicatory (liṅgamātra) non-existent or non-indicatory (aliṅgāni)||19||

There are four states of the primary inherited qualities of elements (gunas), and these are: 1) specialised, or particularised (visheṣa), 2) non-specialised, or non-particularised (avisheṣa), 3) indicator-only, or marked only (linga-matra), and 4) without indicator, or without mark (alingani).

द्रष्टा दृशिमात्रः शुद्धोऽपि प्रत्ययानुपश्यः ॥२०॥
Draṣṭā dṛashi-mātraḥ shuddho api pratyaya-anupashyaḥ||20||

The Seer or perceiver (draṣṭā) is only or merely (mātraḥ) a witness or experiencer (dṛashi) who although (api) pure, untouched or un-effected (shuddhaḥ), experiences (anupaśyaḥ) the mental modifications (pratyaya)||20||

The Seer or Self-Awareness which experiences everything is only the witness of what is to be seen and the force of seeing itself, appearing to experience or see that which is presented as a cognitive principle. This is also mentioned in Bhagavat Gita that our True-Self or Atman is free of all the changes and experiences we go through. Lord Krishna further mentions that "Atman is eternal and untouched of any impurities at all levels."

तदर्थ एव दृश्यस्यात्मा ॥२१॥

Tadartha eva dṛashyasya-ātmā||21||

The True-Nature or essence (ātmā) of the knowable or experience (dṛashyasya) is really (eva) *only one to be known or experienced* (arthaḥ) of That Soul or Purusha (tad)||21||

The essence or nature of the knowing or experiencing objects is only to be used as an instrument or the objective field for knowing or seeing pure consciousness (self-realisation).

कृतार्थं प्रति नष्टमप्यनष्टं तदन्यसाधारणत्वात् ॥२२॥

Kṛata-arthaṁ prati naṣṭam-api-anaṣṭaṁ tad-anya-sādhāra-ṇatvāt||22||

Even though (api) disappeared (naṣṭam) with regard (prati) to the One *(Puruṣa)* who has attained his highest goal or purpose (kṛata-artham), that Atman or True Nature (tad) does not disappear (anaṣṭam) because of being common, all-one or eternal (sādhāra-ṇatvāt) to others (anya) ||22||

Reality or objects and their existence or true nature and real experience is not seen or observed by those who are seeing the gross forms, however their qualities, true nature and fundamentals are still there. Its like if we cant experience or see the true qualities of objects and beings, it does not mean they don't exist, and it's common in the evolutionary path in the beginning where we see only the gross aspects.

स्वस्वामिशक्त्योः स्वरूपोपलब्धिहेतुः संयोगः॥२३॥
Sva-svāmi-shaktyoḥ svarūpa-upalabdhi-hetuḥ
sṁayogaḥ||23||

Union (sṁayogaḥ) is the cause (hetuḥ) for realizing (upalabdhi) the true nature (sva-rūpa) of the two powers (shaktyoḥ) object that exist (sva) master or owner (svāmi)||23||

A union, or attachment between objects and the Self is the root cause of the self being identified with the material and unreal. We may identify ourselves with our body, mind, possessions, etc, but all those are merely instruments or objects.

तस्य हेतुरविद्या॥२४॥
Tasya hetur-avidyā||24||

Ignorance (avidyā) is the cause (hetuḥ) of that *union or attachment with objects* (tasya)||24||

Avidya or ignorance is the root cause of this alliance of Self with matter or the unreal. Avidya is lack of knowing or awareness. Avidya is also denying the truth we know as well as advocating that we know or we are realised when we are not??. In Bhagavat Gita Krishna says that Avidya or ignorance is seeing the objects which are subject to change as Reality and seeing Atman or Soul as subject to all that is not real."

तदभावात्संयोगाभावो हानं तद्दृशेः कैवल्यम् ॥२५॥
Tad-abhāvāt-smayoga-abhāvo hānaṁ tad-dṛasheḥ kaivalyam||25||

The absence (abhāvaḥ) of union or attachment (smayoga) arising from the absence (abhāvāt) of that Avidya or ignorance (tad) is Kaivalya (kaivalyam) or the state of realisation (hānam) of that (tad) *Highest* Witnessing Awareness (dṛasheḥ) *known as Atman, Puruṣa or Soul* ||25||

This means removing the avidya or ignorance leading us in to union with objects or unreality and True Self and detachment from objects through awareness or Vidya (knowledge of Truth or eternity or Purusha or Atman) one attains the highest state of freedom, self-realisation or liberation known as Kaivalyam.

विवेकख्यातिरविप्लवा हानोपायः ॥२६॥
Viveka-khyātir-aviplavā hāna-upāyaḥ||26||

The means or path (upāyaḥ) of Liberation (hāna) is discriminative (viveka) knowledge (khyātiḥ) which is absolutely free of confusion and manipulation (aviplavā)||26||

Clear, uninterrupted, discriminative awareness is the means of liberation from this union or attachment of self with the material.

तस्य सप्तधा प्रान्तभूमिः प्रज्ञा ॥२७॥

Tasya saptadhā prāntabhūmiḥ prajñā||27||

A seven-fold (saptadhā) *and* ultimate or highest (prāntabhūmiḥ) true wisdom (prajñā) is attained by Yogi (tasya)||27||

Seven kinds of ultimate wisdom or knowledge or Samadhi are attained to one who has attained discrimination.

योगाङ्गानुष्ठानादशुद्धिक्षये ज्ञानदीप्तिराविवेकख्यातेः ॥२८॥

Yoga-aṅga-anuṣṭhānād-ashuddhi-kṣaye jñāna-dīptih-ā-viveka-khyāteḥ||28||

On the removal (kṣaye) of impurity (ashuddhi) through the practice or sadhana (anuṣṭhānāt) of the limbs (aṅga) of Yoga (yoga), *one attains* the Light (dīptiḥ) of Wisdom (jñāna) leading (ā) to discriminative (viveka) knowledge (khyāteḥ)||28||

Through the practice of the different limbs, or steps to Yoga, one can purify or remove impurities which will lead Sadhaka to attain discrimination, wisdom, or enlightenment.

यमनियमासनप्राणायामप्रत्याहारधारणाध्यानसमाधयोऽष्टावङ्गानि ॥२९॥

Yama-niyama-āsana-prāṇāyāma-pratyāhāra-dhāraṇā-dhyāna-samādhayo-aṣṭau-aṅgāni||29||

Yama (yama), Niyama (niyama), Āsana (āsana), Prāṇāyāma (prāṇāyāma), Pratyāhāra (pratyāhāra), Dhāraṇā (dhāraṇā), Dhyāna (dhyāna) Samādhi (samādhayo) *are* the eight (aṣṭau) limbs *of Yoga* (aṅgāni) ||29||

The eight limbs, or steps of Yoga are the code of conduct of self-regulation or restraint (yama), observances or practices of self-training (niyama), posture (āsana), expansion of breath and prana (prānāyāma), withdrawal of the senses (pratyāhāra), concentration (dharanā), meditation (dhyāna), and union, liberation (samādhi).

अहिंसासत्यास्तेयब्रह्मचर्यापरिग्रहा यमाः ॥३०॥

Ahiṁsā-satya-asteya-brahmachariya-aparigrahā yamāḥ||30||

Non-injury or non-harm (ahiṁsā), Honesty or truthfulness (satya), non-stealing (asteya), living in harmony with divine creative force (brahmachariya) and Non-possession or taking what is necessary (aparigrahāḥ) *are the five* Yamas or Restraints (yamāḥ)||30||

Non-injury or non-harming (ahimsā), truthfulness, honesty (satya), abstention from stealing or not taking anything that does not belong to us (asteya), living with the laws of nature, sexual or energy discipline (brahmachariya), and non-possessiveness or non-greed (aparigraha) are the five yamās.

जातिदेशकालसमयानवच्छिन्नाः सार्वभौमा महाव्रतम् ॥३१॥

Jāti-desha-kāla-samaya-anavacchinnāḥ sārvabhaumā mahā-vratam||31||

These Yamas are the greatest (mahā) virtues (vratam) *when practised* universally (sārvabhaumāḥ) and all the time without breaking these virtues (anavacchinnāḥ) due to class (jāti), place (desha), time (kāla) or customary duty or obligation (samaya)||31||

These yamas become the great virtues when they are practiced universally and are not restricted or limited to nature or any kind of living being, cast or creed, nor are restricted to any place, time or situation. These virtues should be practised in all situations and not just as and when it is suitable for us.

शौचसन्तोषतपःस्वाध्यायेश्वरप्रणिधानानि नियमाः ॥३२॥

Shaucha-santoṣa-tapaḥ-svādhyāya-ishvara-praṇidhānāni niyamāḥ||32||

Cleanliness or purity (Shauca), Contentment (santoṣa), Austerity or Penance (tapas), Self-Study or introspection and study of scriptures (svādhyāya), and Devotion or faith (praṇidhānāni) in the Divine (īśvara) *are the five* Niyamas or Observances (niyamāḥ)||32||

Cleanliness and purity (shaucha), contentment (santosha), austerity, practice (tapas), self-study and reflection (svādhyāya), and perceiving life and every moment as a divine blessing (ishvara-prashādhana or praṇidhānāni) are the observances or Niyamas.

वितर्कबाधने प्रतिपक्षभावनम् ॥३३॥
Vitarka-bādhane pratipakṣa-bhāvanam||33||

On the inhibition (bādhane) of Yamas and Niyamas due to negative thoughts and feelings, A Yogi should contemplate (bhāvanam) on the opposites (pratipakṣa)||33||

Think or contemplate on opposite thoughts of principles, when you feel disturbed or deviated from adhering to yamās and niyamās due to troublesome thoughts. In this sutra Patanjali explains one of the most simple and profound solution to all those negative forces, thoughts and feelings leading us into non-virtuous behaviour. He says, "Focus your mind or positive or higher thoughts- which are opposite to negative or lower ones."

वितर्का हिंसादयः कृतकारितानुमोदिता लोभक्रोधमोहपूर्वका मृदुमध्याधिमात्रा दुःखाज्ञानानन्तफला इति प्रतिपक्षभावनम् ॥३४॥
Vitarkā hiṁsādayaḥ kṛata-kārita-anumoditā lobha-krodha-moha-pūrvakā mṛadu-madhya-adhimātrā duḥkha-ajñāna-ananta-phalā iti pratipakṣa-bhāvanam||34||

Such non-virtuous actions like injury (hiṁsā), and all other ways (ādayaḥ) resulting from negative or irrational thinking or feelings (vitarkāḥ) are those 1. which are performed by oneself (kṛata), getting them done by others by any means (kārita) or approved or allowed (anumoditāḥ); ***2.*** those which are caused or resulted (pūrvakāḥ) by greed (lobha), anger (krodha), or delusion (moha). *These actions can be* mild (mṛadu), moderate (madhya) or intense (adhimātrāḥ) in intensity. They are unending (ananta) of fruits or consequences (phalāḥ) *resulting from* pain (duḥkha) *and* ignorance (ajñāna)" for the remedy of all the above practise contemplation on the opposite (pratipakṣa-bhāvanam)||34||

Actions under influence of negative thoughts are performed directly by oneself, caused to be done through others in any means, or being approved when done by others. All of these may be influenced by, or performed due to anger, greed or delusion, and can be mild, moderate or intense in nature. These thoughts and actions lead to ignorance and miseries and the remedy is thinking on or contemplating on the the opposite as/of? above sutra. This Sutra explains that we should always keep contemplating, reflecting and practising Yamas and Niyamas at all levels- thoughts, feelings, speech and actions.

अहिंसाप्रतिष्ठायां तत्सन्निधौ वैरत्यागः॥३५॥

Ahiṁsā-pratiṣṭhāyāṁ tat-sannidhau vaira-tyāgaḥ||35||

On the mastery in practice (pratiṣṭhāyām) of Ahiṁsā or Non-violence (ahiṁsā) *there is* cessation or absence (tyāgaḥ) of hostility or enmity (vaira) by anyone coming close (sannidhau) to him/her (tad)||35||

When one masters non-violence (ahimsa), all others abandon enmity or hostilities around them.

सत्यप्रतिष्ठायां क्रियाफलाश्रयत्वम् ॥३६॥

Satya-pratiṣṭhāyāṁ kriya-phal-āshrayatvam||36||

On the mastery(pratiṣṭhāyām) of Satya or Truthfulness (satya) a state of connection or oneness (āśrayatvam) between *his* actions (kriyā) and the fruits or consequences (phala) *is attained.* ||36||

As truthfulness (satya) is mastered in practice, one acquires all the fruits of actions according to their own will.

अस्तेयप्रतिष्ठायां सर्वरत्नोपस्थानम् ॥३७॥

Asteya-pratiṣṭhāyāṁ sarva-ratna-upasthānam||37||

On the mastery (pratiṣṭhāyām) of Asteya or Non-stealing (asteya) all (sarva) jewels (ratna) are attained or gained (upasthānam) by Yogi||37||

When non-stealing (asteya) is mastered in practice, all jewels, or treasures and wealth follow the Yogi. This is a state of living in true abundance of happiness with all the material possession one has? desire of as a Sadhaka has mastered the state of not taking anything that does not belong to him.

ब्रह्मचर्यप्रतिष्ठायां वीर्यलाभः ॥३८॥

Brahmachariya-pratiṣṭhāyāṁ vīriya-lābhaḥ||38||

On the mastery (pratiṣṭhāyām) of life energy discipline (brahmachariya) *the Yogi* acquires (lābhaḥ) the energy, vigour, vitality, strength (vīrya)||38||

Mastery of Brahmachariya or Discipline of energy and actions lead to vitality, health and well-being.

अपरिग्रहस्थैर्ये जन्मकथन्तासम्बोधः ॥३९॥

Aparigraha-sthairye janma-kathantā-sambodhaḥ||39||

When *one follows* firmly (sthairye) the Non-possession (aparigraha), complete knowledge (sambodhaḥ) of existence or birth about "how, what state in context to past, present and future (janma-kathantā) *is known*||39||

Mastery of non-greed (aparigraha), one acquires knowledge of past and future incarnations.

शौचात्स्वाङ्गजुगुप्सा परैरसंसर्गः ॥४०॥

Shauchāt-sva-aṅga-jugupsā paraih-asaṁsargaḥ||40||

From mastering the Shauca or Purity (Shauchāt), detachment (jugupsā) from one›s own (sva) body (aṅga) is mastered and it leads into non-attraction or freedom from any concerns to contact (asaṁsargaḥ) with others (paraiḥ) ||40||

Through cleanliness and purity of body and mind (shaucha), one develops detachment from one's own body as well as any attachment or attraction towards other's bodies or possessions.

सत्त्वशुद्धिसौमनस्यैकाग्र्येन्द्रियजयात्मदर्शनयोग्यत्वानि च॥४१॥

Sattva-shuddhi-saumanasya-ekāgriya-indriya-jayātma-darshana-yogyatvāni cha||41||

Along with purity (shuddhi) of the subtlest of primary nature (sattva), mental satisfaction (saumanasya), single-pointedness (aikāgriya), mastery (jaya) of the senses (5 Jñānendriyas or of organs of cognition and 5 Karmendriyas or organs of action) (indriya) *and* ability (yogyatvāni) for perceiving or realising (darshana) the Self (ātma), *are* also (cha) *attained* ||41||

Also cleanliness and purity of body and mind (shaucha) brings purification of the subtle primary qualities or essence (sattva), a pleasantness, happiness in feeling, a single-pointedness and awareness in everything one does, mastery over the senses, and gains fitness, qualification, or capability for self-realisation.

सन्तोषादनुत्तमसुखलाभः॥४२॥

Santoṣāt-anuttama-sukha-lābhaḥ||42||

From mastery of Contentment (santoṣāt); *there is abundance* (lābhaḥ) of infinite or divine (anuttama) happiness (sukha)||42||

Eternal happiness, mental balance, joy, and satisfaction are obtained from mastering contentment or santoṣa.

कायेन्द्रियसिद्धिरशुद्धिक्षयात्तपसः ॥४३॥

Kāya-indriya-siddhih-ashuddhi-kṣayāt-tapasaḥ||43||

For Perfection or mastery (siddhiḥ) of the body (kāya) and senses (5 Jñānendriyas, and 5 Karmendriyas) (indriya) *is attained* through Tapas or Austerity (tapasaḥ), which removes or purifies (kṣayāt) impurities (aśuddhi)||43||

One can master or perfect the body, and senses, through dedicated practice of austerity as well as to remove all the impurities of body, mind, emotions, intellect, one must follow the right practices or path of austerity known as Tapas.

स्वाध्यायादिष्टदेवतासम्प्रयोगः ॥४४॥

Svādhyāyāt-iṣṭa-devatā-samprayogaḥ||44||

Union or communion (samprayogaḥ) with the desired or chosen (iṣṭa) deity (devatā) *is attained* from Svādhyāya or Self-Study and Study of Sacred Scriptures (svādhyāyāt)||44||

From the study of scripture, contemplations of these great teachings, self-study and introspection (svādhyāya), one attains communion, or union with the divine force or eternal real-self.

समाधिसिद्धिरीश्वरप्रणिधानात् ॥४५॥

Samādhi-siddhih-īshvara-praṇidhānāt||45||

Perfection or mastery (siddhiḥ) of Samādhi or Union or Self-realisation (samādhi) *is attained* through devotion, faith and dedication (praṇidhānāt) in divine creative force (īshvara)||45||

From an attitude and perception of seeing divine reality of every event as a blessing and dedicating our life, all actions, thoughts and feelings to divine cause leads to enlightenment, liberation, or samadhi.

स्थिरसुखमासनम् ॥४६॥

Sthirasukhamāsanam||46||

A firm (sthira) and pleasant or comfortable (sukham) seat is āsana (āsanam) ||46||

A steady, stable or motionless, position with comfort or ease is known as āsana or posture. This is the highest state of our being at ease or comfort with our own body, mind and soul.

प्रयत्नशैथिल्यानन्तसमापत्तिभ्याम् ॥४७॥

Prayatna-shaithilya-ananta-samāpattibhyām||47||

Through continuous letting go of effort (prayatna) by means of relaxation or ease (shaithilya) one attains a deep state of awareness or samadhi known as samāpatti (samāpattibhyām) in the infinite (ananta), Asana is perfected ||47||

Practice repeatedly and regularly with relaxing and letting go of effort with engaging or focussing our mind on the eternal or infinite will lead to mastery of āsana.

ततो द्वन्द्वानभिघातः ॥४८॥

Tato dvandva-anabhighātaḥ||48||

From that (tato), *one remains un-effected* (anabhighātaḥ) when facing the pairs of opposites (dvandva)||48||

Mastering the āsana brings freedom from disturbances, sufferings caused by duality or pairs of two opposites like pain-pleasure, like-dislike, hot-cold.

तस्मिन्सति श्वासप्रश्वासयोर्गतिविच्छेदः
प्राणायामः ॥४९॥

Tasmin-sati shvāsa-prashvāsayoh-gati-vicchedaḥ
prāṇāyāmaḥ||49||

Once that (tasmin) *Āsana* has been mastered (sati), Prāṇāyāma (prāṇāyāmaḥ), which is the retention or extension (vicchedaḥ) of the flow (gati) of inhalation (shvāsa) and exhalation- (prashvāsayoḥ), *should be followed* ||49||

Once āsana or posture is perfected, retaining or expanding the inhaling and exhaling of breath for expansion and retention of prana known as **prāṇāyāma** should be practised.

वाह्याभ्यन्तरस्तम्भवृत्तिः देशकालसङ्ख्याभिः परिदृष्टो
दीर्घसूक्ष्मः ॥५०॥

Bāhya-abhyantara-stambha-vṛattih-desha-kāla-
saṅkhyābhiḥ pari-dṛaṣṭo dīrgha-sūkṣmaḥ||50||

Prāṇāyāma has *(three)* parts (vṛattiḥ):
1. External (bāhya),
2. Internal (ābhyantara) and ***3.*** Retention (stambha).
When Prāṇāyāma is followed (paridṛṣṭaḥ) according to space (desha), time (kāla) and number (saṅkhyābhiḥ), it becomes long (dīrgha) and subtle (sūkṣmaḥ)||50||

That **prāṇāyāma** has three aspects, the out breath or exhalation, the in breath or inhalation and the third aspect is retention or resting of inhaling and exhaling breath. These are mastered in place, time, number or rhythms with breath becoming slow, deep and subtle.

वाह्याभ्यन्तरविषयाक्षेपी चतुर्थः॥५१॥

Bāhya-abhyantara-viṣaya-akṣepī chaturthaḥ||51||

The fourth *type of Prāṇāyāma* (chaturthaḥ) transcends or goes beyond (ākṣepī) the subjects of influence (viṣaya) of External (Bāhya) and Internal (ābhyantara) activities or operations ||51||

The fourth **prāṇāyāma** is that eternal or subtle prana which transcends, and is beyond, or behind those others, operating in the form of the exterior and interior realms or fields.

ततः क्षीयते प्रकाशावरणम्॥५२॥

Tataḥ kṣīyate prakāsha-avaraṇam||52||

Through that (tata), the veil or layers (āvaraṇam) over Prakāsha or light of true wisdom (prakāsha) is cleared or removed (kṣīyate)||52||

The mastery of **prāṇāyāma** removes or clears the shield or covering of karma, etc from the eternal or inner illumination or light and wisdom.

धारणासु च योग्यता मनसः॥५३॥

Dhāraṇāsu cha yogyatā manasaḥ||53||

Mental (manasaḥ) fitness or ability (yogyatā) focus or concentrate (dhāraṇāsu) *is* also (cha) *developed*||53||

Capability, ability or qualification of mind to focus on one point is also attained by **prāṇāyāma**.

स्वविषयासम्प्रयोगे चित्तस्य स्वरूपानुकार इवेन्द्रियाणां प्रत्याहारः ॥५४॥

Sva-viṣaya-asamprayoge chittasya svarūpa-anukāra iva-indriyāṇāṁ pratyāhāraḥ||54||

The Withdrawal (pratyāhāraḥ) of senses (indriyāṇām) *is* as if they (iva), are following (anukāraḥ) the essential nature (sva-rūpa) of the mind (chittasya) when separated (asamprayoge) from their *corresponding* (sva) objects of experiences (viṣaya)||54||

When the senses (in yoga cognitive and action senses-indriyas) are not engaged with the corresponding external objects or stimulus in their mental realm, and instead engaged inward into the mind-field from which they arose this is the fifth limb known as pratyāhāra.

ततः परमा वश्यतेन्द्रियाणाम् ॥५५॥

Tataḥ paramā vaśyatendriyāṇām||55||

From that *Pratyāhāra* (tatas), supreme (paramā) mastery or control (vaśyatā) of the experiences actions of sense organs (indriyāṇām) *is attained* ||55||

Through this sensory withdrawal or introversion one masters the senses and their actions either to go inward or outwards.

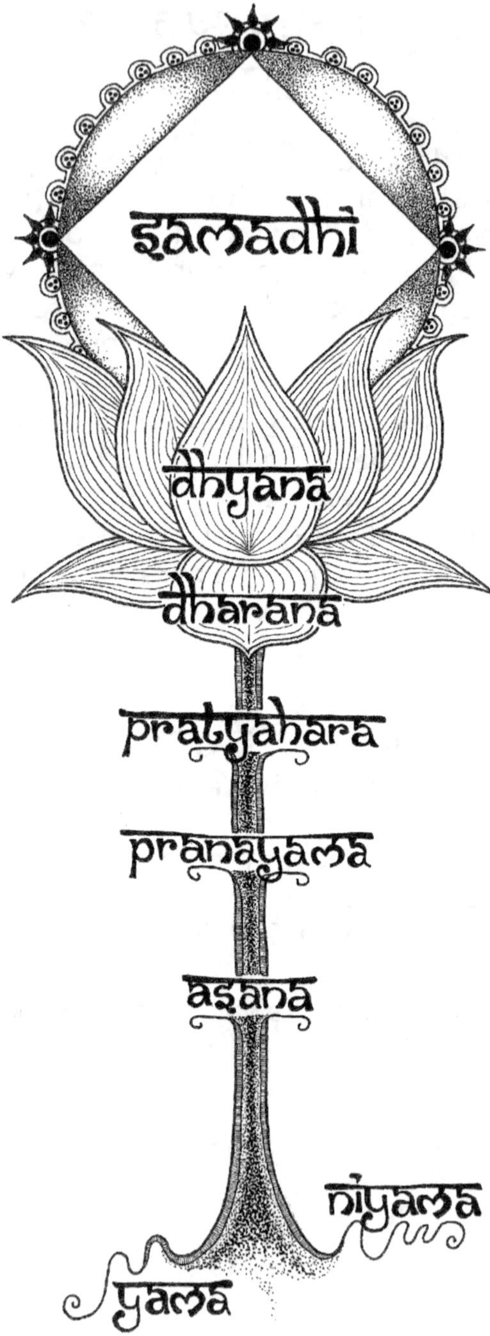
samadhi
dhyana
dharana
pratyahara
pranayama
asana
niyama
yama

Chapter 3 : Vibhuti Pāda

देशबन्धश्चित्तस्य धारणा ॥१॥
Desha-bandhah-chittasya dhāraṇā||1||

Concentration (dhāraṇā) is the mind›s (chittasya) undisturbed focus (bandhaḥ) on a single point (desha)||1||

Dharana is the 6th limb of Ashtānga yoga. Dharanā or Concentration is the process of holding or focussing the awareness or mind on one object or point.

तत्र प्रत्ययैकतानता ध्यानम् ॥२॥
Tatra pratyaya-ekatānatā dhyānam||2||

In that concentration or dharnā (tatra), the continuous and long single pointed (ekatānatā) outcome of absorption of mind in that one point (pratyaya) is Meditation (dhyānam)||2||

From effort to focussing our mind on a single-point of concentration, when the mind or awareness is completely absorbed in that one point or object of concentration it is known as dhyān or meditation. This is the 7th limb of ashtanga yoga.

तदेवार्थमात्रनिर्भासं स्वरूपशून्यमिव समाधिः ॥३॥

Tad-eva-artha-mātra-nirbhāsaṁ svarūpa-shūnyam-iva samādhiḥ||3||

Ultimate Union or the highest state of awareness (samādhiḥ) is just (eva) that *state* (tad) in which only (mātra) the object or point of *concentration* (artha) remains in focus (nirbhāsam), and the self-identity (sva-rūpa) is absent or dissolved (shūnyam), as it were (iva) the focus point itself ||3||

When the mind is completely absorbed in the object, point, or form of concentration or its meaning and loses its identity with itself it is known as samadhi or enlightenment. This is the 8th limb of ashtanga yoga.

त्रयमेकत्र संयमः ॥४॥

Trayam-ekatra saṁyamaḥ||4||

These three (Dhāraṇā, Dhyāna and Samādhi) (trayam) all together on one point (ekatra) are known as Saṁyama (higher or internal yoga) (saṁyamaḥ)||4||

Dharanā, dhyāna, and samādhi, all three are practiced together on single point, object or concept and is known as samyama or higher yoga.

तज्जयात्प्रज्ञालोकः ॥५॥

Tad-jayāt-prajñā-ālokaḥ||5||

Through the mastery (jayāt) of that Sṁayama (tad), the Light (ālokaḥ) of Wisdom (prajñā) *manifests or dawns* ||5||

Inner light, transcendental awareness or higher consciousness awakens or illuminates by mastering Samayama.

तस्य भूमिषु विनियोगः ॥६॥

Tasya bhūmiṣu viniyogaḥ||6||

These must be followed or practised (viniyogaḥ) of that (tasya) to the stages in the order *of the practice* (bhūmiṣu)||6||

That three-fold awareness in practice of samyama is gradually applied to the all stages of practice in the order of concentration, meditation and samadhi.

त्रयमन्तरङ्गं पूर्वेभ्यः॥७॥

Trayam-antar-aṅgaṁ pūrvebhyaḥ||7||

These three (trayam) *are the* internal *limbs* (antar-aṅgam) compared to the previous limbs of yoga, i.e. Yama, Niyama, Āsana, Prāṇāyāma and Pratyāhāra (pūrvebhyaḥ) ||7||

These three concentration, meditation, and samadhi are internal limbs of the higher limbs of yoga compared to the previous five limbs- yama, niyama, asana, pranayama and pratyahara.

तदपि वहिरङ्गं निर्वीजस्य॥८॥

Tad-api bahir-aṅgaṁ nirbījasya||8||

These three (tad api) are the external limbs (bahir-aṅgam) in comparison or respect of Nirbīja or seedless concentration (nirbījasya)||8||

However, these three limbs are external, and not internal compared to nirbija samadhi. Samādhi that has no object, or a seed of concentration is Nirbija Samādhi.

व्युत्थाननिरोधसंस्कारयोरभिभवप्रादुर्भावौ
निरोधक्षणचित्तान्वयो निरोधपरिणामः॥९॥

Vyutthāna-nirodha-saṁskārayoh-abhibhava-prādurbhāvau nirodha-kṣaṇa-chitta-anvayah nirodha-pariṇāmaḥ||9||

The dissolving or clearing (abhibhava) of the latent impressions (saṁskārayoḥ) of their rising (vyutthāna) and the appearance or manifestation (prādurbhāvau) of the subtle impressions (saṁskārayoḥ) of a mastered or peaceful state of mind (nirodha) *is* the result of fruit (pariṇāmaḥ) of a *mastered or pure* state of mind (nirodha). *This outcome or fruit* is linked (anvayaḥ) to the mind (chitta) at *every* moment (kṣaṇa) of that mastered or purest state of mind (nirodha)||9||

Deep or highest Samadhi or Nirodha occurs in that moment when arousing subtle impressions and dissolving subtle impressions are dissolved into the consciousness itself.

तस्य प्रशान्तवाहिता संस्कारात्॥१०॥

Tasya prashānta-vāhitā saṁskārāt||10||

Through these latent impressions (saṁskārāt) of that mastered state of mind (tasya), an unbroken and undisturbed state of mental peace or equanimity (prashānta-vāhitā) *is attained* ||10||

By keeping our mind absorbed or focussed on these subtle impressions or Samaskaras of that state of union, peace or tranquil mind, that state of mastered mind or peaceful mind becomes unbroken, undisturbed and ever-lasting.

सर्वार्थतैकाग्रतयोः क्षयोदयौ चित्तस्य
समाधिपरिणामः॥११॥
Sarva-arthatā-ekāgratayoḥ kṣaya-udayau chittasya
samādhi-pariṇāmaḥ||11||

Removal or clearing (kṣaya) of attachment of
all objects (sarva-arthatā) and the development
(udayau) of single-pointedness (ekāgratayoḥ) *is* the
result (pariṇāmaḥ) Highest Awareness or
Union (samādhi) of the mind (chittasya)||11||

Samadhi occurs when all or many-pointedness and single pointedness dissolves into consciousness or the purest form of mind.

ततः पुनः शान्तोदितौ तुल्यप्रत्ययौ
चित्तस्यैकाग्रतापरिणामः॥१२॥
Tataḥ punaḥ shānta-uditau tulya-pratyayau chittasya-
ekāgratā-pariṇāmaḥ||12||

There in state of Samadhi (tatas) again (punah)
the quietened (shānta) modifications
(pratyayau) being the same (tulya) as the present
arising (uditau) modifications (pratyayau),
result (pariṇāmaḥ) in the single-pointed
awareness (ekāgratā) of the mind (chittasya)||12||

Then again through mastering single-pointed awareness and absorbing quietening and arising modifications in the mind field or chitta, one achieves mastery of the state of single-pointedness (ekagrata-parinamah) or Samadhi.

एतेन भूतेन्द्रियेषु धर्मलक्षणावस्थापरिणामा व्याख्याताः॥१३॥

Etena bhūta-indriyeṣu dharma-lakṣaṇa-avasthā-pariṇāmā vyākhyātāḥ||13||

By means of those (etena), results or fruits of single-pointedness (pariṇāmāḥ) of true and eternal qualities or attributions (dharma), active or observable character (lakṣana) state of being (avasthā) in the fundamental elements (earth, water, air, fire and ether) (bhūta) and organs of cognitive actions (indriyeṣu) are known or experienced in detail (vyākhyātāḥ)||13||

During these three states or results in the form of single-pointed awareness of Samadhi and their processes, one also achieves knowledge or experience of the form, time, and characteristics, and how these are produced through the senses.

शान्तोदिताव्यपदेश्यधर्मानुपाती धर्मी॥१४॥

Shānta-udita-avyapadeshya-dharma-anupātī dharmī||14||

The inherited characters (dharmī) continue to exist (anupātī) through characteristics in the form of (dharma): dissolved or past (śānta), manifest or present (udita) and indefinable, once yet to manifest, or future (avyapadeśya)||14||

The quietening and arising of chitta is continuously followed as those characters are inherited with the objects to chitta and these can be in one of three forms- 1. quietened or ones which are past, 2. manifest, arising, active, of present and 3. Unknown, yet to manifest or future.

क्रमान्यत्वं परिणामान्यत्वे हेतुः॥१५॥

Krama-anyatvaṁ pariṇāma-anyatve hetuḥ||15||

Difference (anyatvam) in the sequence or order (krama) *is* the cause (hetuḥ) of the difference (anyatve) in the result (pariṇāma) in ||15||

Change in the sequence of experiences of the objects and their characters is the cause for the different results, fruits or siddhis.

परिणामत्रयसंयमादतीतानागतज्ञानम्॥१६॥

Pariṇāma-traya-saṁyamāt-atīta-anāgata-jñānam||16||

Knowledge (jñānam) of past (atīta) *and* future (anāgata) *is attained* through Dhārnā, Dhyāna and Samādhi (saṁyamāt) on the three (traya) as a result or fruit (pariṇāma) ||16||

There comes knowledge of the past and future, by mastering samyama on three levels- **Dhārnā** (concentration), **Dhyāna** (meditation), and **Samādhi** together.

शब्दार्थप्रत्ययानामितरेतराध्यासात्सङ्करस्तत्प्रविभागसंयमात्सर्वभूतरुतज्ञानम् ॥१७॥

Shabda-artha-pratyayānām-itaretara-adhyāsāt-saṅkarah-tat-pravibhāga-saṁyamāt-sarvabhūta-ruta-jñānam||17||

Through the above (itaretara) overlaying or superimposing (adhyāsāt) of word (shabda), meaning (artha) *and* idea or concept (pratyayānām), a mixture of these above appearing as if they are one (saṅkaraḥ) *is known or identified by* mastering the last three limbs of Yoga (saṁyamāt) on that *(mix of word, meaning and idea)* (tad), but saperately (pravibhāga), knowledge (jñānam)of *the true essence* (ruta) *all-pervading* (sarva) in beings that which exist (bhūta) *is acquired*||17||

The name, sound or word, meaning and concepts associated with the objects are overlaying or superimposed with one and other. By mastering samyāma one achieves knowledge of all the elements, their sounds, meanings and their concepts.

संस्कारसाक्षात्करणात्पूर्वजातिज्ञानम् ॥१८॥

Saṁskāra-sākṣātkaraṇāt-pūrva-jāti-jñānam||18||

Knowledge (jñānam) of previous (pūrva) births (jāti) *is acquired* through the realisation (sākṣātkaraṇāt) of latent subtle impressions (saṁskāra)||18||

Through the direct perception of subtle impressions or deep rooted belief systems (saṁskāra) one attains knowledge of the previous births or incarnations.

प्रत्ययस्य परचित्तज्ञानम् ॥१९॥
Pratyayasya para-chitta-jñānam||19||

Knowledge (jñānam) of the others› minds (para-citta) *is acquired by mastering Samayāma* on the notions or ideas presented (pratyayasya)||19||

By *Samayāma* on the notions or presented ideas one attains the siddhi to know another's mind.

न च तत्सालम्बनं तस्याविषयीभूतत्वात् ॥२०॥
Na cha tat-sālambanaṁ tasya-aviṣayī-bhūtatvāt||20||

The foundation of support of (sālambanam) of those notions or ideas (tad) certainly (ca) is not (na) attained from Samyama because it is (bhūtatvāt) out of experience or reach (aviṣayī) of him (tasya) ||20||

But that Being-ness or the consciousness is not experienced because is beyond reach of sensory experience even of a Yogi.

कायरूपसंयमात्तद्ग्राह्यशक्तिस्तम्भेचक्षुःप्रकाशासम्प्रयोगेऽन्तर्धानम्॥२१॥

Kāya-rūpa-saṁyamāt-tad-grāhya-shakti-stambhe cakṣuḥ-prakāsha-asamprayoge-antardhānam||21||

On power or ability of holding or establishing (shakti-stambhe) of perception and experiencing (grāhya) of that body (tad) through Saṁyama (saṁyamāt) on the form and qualities (rūpa) of the body (kāya), and when the Yogī is free of any attachment or experience of the body (asamprayoge) divine light or awareness is attained (chakṣuḥ-prakāsha), where the *mind absorbs in that inner meditation* (antardhānam)||21||

When samyama is practiced on the form of one's own physical body, one achieves the capacity to perceive the light or visual characteristics or knowledge which are invisible to our eyes. This is also known as astral access where one can access the cosmic knowledge or wisdom. Here one has to go beyond the body through meditating on it and gradually letting the physical body and absorb the awareness in light or vital forces (shakti-stambhe).

सोपक्रमं निरुपक्रमं च कर्म
तत्संयमादपरान्तज्ञानमरिष्टेभ्यो वा ॥२२॥

Sopakramaṁ nirupakramaṁ cha karma tat-saṁyamāt-aparānta-jñānam-ariṣṭebhyo vā||22||

Karma or action (karma) *is of two kinds* 1. Fruiting or resulting instantly (sopakramam) and (cha) fruiting or resulting sometime later (nirupakramam). By practising Saṁyama (saṁyamāt) on *karma* (tad) or (vā) one attains knowledge (jñānam) death and its time (aparānta) before it happens (ariṣṭebhyaḥ)||22||

Karma is of two kinds 1. instant Karma to fruit immediately after action and 2. bija-karma which is to fruit or bring results later in life. Through samyama on these karmas one gains knowledge of the death and time of death before it happens.

मैत्र्यादिषु बलानि ॥२३॥

Maitryā-ādiṣu balāni||23||

Through Saṁyama on friendliness (maitryā) and so on (ādiṣu), one acquires strengths (balāni) ||23||

By samyama on friendliness and others (maitri, karunā, muditā, upekshā (Yoga Sutra 1.33), there comes great strength or power. This sutra explains the strength of unity and collectiveness. When we live with these great virtues, we attain friendship and harmony with all and everyone and hence our strength multiplies.

बलेषु हस्तिबलादीनि ॥२४॥
Baleṣu hasti-balādīni||24||

By mastering Saṁyama on strengths (baleṣu), the strength (bala) of an elephant (hasti), and others (ādīni) *is attained* ||24||

By samyama on the strength one achieves strengths of or like elephants. This strength of knowing or awareness of our abilities, skills and power which is abundance of self-worth and will power.

प्रवृत्त्यालोकन्यासात्सूक्ष्मव्यवहितविप्रकृष्टज्ञानम् ॥२५॥
Pravṛittyah-aloka-nyāsāt-sūkṣma-vyavahita-viprakṛṣṭa-jñānam||25||

By directing (nyāsāt) the inner light (āloka) of the higher sensory (pravṛtti), knowledge (jñānam) of the subtle (sūkṣma), *which are hidden or not experienced* from (vyavahita) *the* remoteness of our external (viprakṛṣṭa), *is obtained)*||25||

By directing the inner light of higher sensory activity, one attains knowledge of subtle objects, those beyond perception or view, and those very distant.

भुवनज्ञानं सूर्ये संयमात्॥२६॥

Bhuvana-jñānaṁ sūrye saṁyamāt||26||

Through Saṁyama (saṁyamāt) on the Sun or the solar energy (sūrye), knowledge (jñānam) of the universe (bhuvana) is attained ||26||

By samyama on the sun or solar energy, knowledge of the whole universe can be known. Our Pranic energy represents Prana, loma, solar or positive energy. By following samayama on this Pranic or solar energy, one will know the universe by knowing itself. It is like a drop of water represents the whole ocean. If one gets to know a drop, one will know the whole ocean. Also our body represents the whole universe. This can be easily understood by understanding the chakra and kundalini system.

चन्द्रे ताराव्यूहज्ञानम्॥२७॥

Chandre tārā-vyūha-jñānam||27||

Through Saṁyama on the moon or lunar energy (chandre), knowledge (jñānam) of the arrangements (vyūha) of stars (tārā) is gained ||27||

By samyama on the moon or lunar energy also known as Apana or Viloma, one masters knowledge of the arrangement of the stars.

ध्रुवे तद्गतिज्ञानम् ॥२८॥

Dhruve tad-gati-jñānam||28||

By mastering Saṁyama on the pole star (dhruve), knowledge (jñānam) of the movement (gati) of those stars (tad) *is attained* ||28||

By samyama on the pole-star, one acquires knowledge of the movement of those stars.

नाभिचक्रे कायव्यूहज्ञानम् ॥२९॥

Nābhi-chakre kaya-vyūha-jñānam||29||

By mastering Saṁyama on the Manipura Chakra or Solar-Plexus (nābhi-chakre), knowledge (jñānam) of the structure and functioning (vyūha) of the body (kāya) *is acquired* ||29||

By samyama on the Manipura Chakra or solar plexus, one masters knowledge about the arrangement of the systems and functions of the body.

कण्ठकूपे क्षुत्पिपासानिवृत्तिः ॥३०॥
Kaṇṭha-kūpe kṣut-pipāsā-nivṛittiḥ||30||

Through mastering Saṁyama on the chakra (kūpe) of the throat (kaṇṭha), *one masters* (nivṛittiḥ) hunger (kṣut) *and* thirst (pipāsā)||30||

By samyama on the throat, one masters hunger and thirst. Our throat area is known as Vishuddha Chakra and is associated with the thyroid gland. This gland regulates our metabolic activities at cellular level and by mastering this chakra, our body will go into a deep state of rest, where metabolic activities will be almost ceased, which explains this Siddhi.

कूर्मनाड्यां स्थैर्यम् ॥३१॥
Kūrma-nāḍyāṁ sthairyam||31||

Through Saṁyama on the naris or channels of breathing (kūrma-nāḍyām), calmness, steadiness and firmness (sthairyam) *is attained* ||31||

By samyama on the Kurma Nari steadiness is attained. Kurma Nari is associated with our inspiration-expiration and physically represented in the bronchial tract. Our irregular breathing is associated with non-stability, agitation, and distress. Samayama on Kurma Nari will lead into deep-conscious and relax breathing, which will bring calmness, ease, and stability.

मूर्धज्योतिषि सिद्धदर्शनम्॥३२॥

Mūrdha-jyotiṣi siddha-darshanam||32||

Saṁyama on the light (jyotiṣi) of the crown (mūrdha) one attains vision or companionship (darshanam) of the Siddhas (siddha)||32||

By samyama on the murdha light (inner light at the crown of the head), one will have visions or companionship of the siddhas, or the masters. This is siddhi where you will have access to all those divine liberated masters. These masters are always there to help and protect us in our Sadhana.

प्रातिभाद्वा सर्वम्॥३३॥

Prātibhād-vā sarvam||33||

Or (vā) through intuitive light of bliss (prātibhāt), everything (sarvam) *is known*||33||

Or, through the intuitive light of bliss, everything will become known. Intuitive bliss is knowledge which comes to a Yogī before the attainment of discriminative knowledge or Viveka.

हृदये चित्तसंवित् ॥३४॥
Hṛadaye chitta-saṁvit||34||

Practice of Saṁyama on the heart (hṛadaye), knowledge (saṁvid) of mind (chitta) *is acquired*||34||

By practicing samyama on the heart, knowledge of the mind or consciousness is attained. Hradaya or Heart centre is known as Anhata Chakra which is the area of our conscious mind or chitta. From here our mind expresses its dynamic-universal-qualities.

सत्त्वपुरुषयोरत्यन्तासङ्कीर्णयोः प्रत्ययाविशेषो भोगः
परार्थत्वात्स्वार्थसंयमात्पुरुषज्ञानम्॥३५॥

Sattva-puruṣayoh-atyanta-asaṅkīrṇayoḥ pratyaya-avisheṣo bhogaḥ parārthatvāt-svārtha-saṁyamāt-puruṣa-jñānam||35||

What we experience (bhogaḥ) *based on* concept or idea (pratyaya) which is there (aviśeṣaḥ) *all the time or* completely (atyanta) is different (asaṅkīrṇayoḥ) *in form of purity or eternity* (sattva) The Real Self or Atman (puruṣayoḥ), exists for the Knower of Yogi (parārthatvāt). Through practising Saṁyama (saṁyamāt) on Puruṣa Higher Self (svārtha), knowledge (jñānam) of Self or Atman (puruṣa) *is obtained*||35||

The experiences of the conscious mind from a presented idea or concept and pure consciousness (purusha), are different. Samyama on the pure consciousness, which is distinct from the subtlest aspect of the mind, reveals knowledge of that pure consciousness. This is awareness of awareness itself. Awareness of what we experience through our mundane mind brings painful or pleasant experiences which is driven by rajas or tamas qualities. While experience from our pure consciousness is driven by sattva or purest of qualities, which is knowledge of our real or higher self.

ततः प्रातिभश्रावणवेदनादर्शास्वादवार्ता जायन्ते॥३६॥
Tataḥ prātibha-shrāvaṇa-vedanā-ādarsha-āsvāda-vārtā jāyante||36||

From that *Saṁyama on Puruṣa or Higher Self* (tatas), intuitive knowledge or light (prātibha), supernatural powers of hearing (shrāvaṇa), touch (vedana), seeing (ādarsha), tasting (āsvāda) *and* smelling (vārtāḥ) arise or awake (jāyante)||36||

From mastering Samayama on Atman of Self one experiences the light of the pure consciousness or purusha through which one attains supernatural, transcendental, or divine powers of hearing, touch, vision, taste, and smell.

ते समाधावुपसर्गा व्युत्थाने सिद्धयः॥३७॥
Te samādhau-upasargā vyutthāne siddhayaḥ||37||

Those *supernormal powers* (te) are obstacles or hindrances (upasargāḥ) in path to Samādhi (samādhau), *but are masteries or fruits of perfection* (siddhayaḥ) for the ordinary mind (vyutthāne)||37||

These experiences resulting from samyama are obstacles to samadhi, but appear to be attainments or powers to the worldly mind which is subject to whirlpools and fluctuations. Here Patanjali is warning Yoga Sadhakas not to get caught in the miracle powers of the mind.

बन्धकारणशैथिल्यात्प्रचारसंवेदनाच्च चित्तस्य परशरीरावेशः॥३८॥

Bandha-kāraṇa-shaithilyāt-prachāra-saṁvedanāt-cha chittasya para-sharīr-āveśaḥ||38||

Through the clearing or removal (śaithilyāt) of the cause (kāraṇa) of bondage or attachment (bandha) and (cha) complete knowledge or understanding (saṁvedanāt) of the roaming (prachāra) of mind (chittasya), *one can enter* (āveshaḥ) into the body (sharīra) of another (para) ||38||

By removing, purifying or letting go the causes of bondage or attachment, and by following the knowledge of how to go forth into the deeper levels of the mind, one masters the ability to enter into another's body.

उदानजयाज्जलपङ्ककण्टकादिष्वसङ्ग उत्क्रान्तिश्च ॥३९॥

Udāna-jayāt-jala-paṅka-kaṇṭak-ādiṣu-asaṅga utkrāntish-cha||39||

By mastering (jayāt) Udana, one of the five pranas (udāna), *one attains mastery from any harm from* (asaṅgaḥ) water (jala), mud (paṅka), thorns (kaṇṭaka), etc. (ādiṣu) and (cha) and will leave the body with will or knowingly at time of death (utkrāntiḥ)||39||

By the mastery over Udana, there is a siddhi or power which keeps Sadhaka aware from any harm or contact from mud, water, thorns, and other such objects, and one achieves levitation of the body. Udana is one of the panch-pranas or subtle vital life forces governing Udana vayu and is located in the throat area and flows in a circular manner around the neck and head. This vayu regulates speech, growth and self-expression.

समानजयाज्ज्वलनम् ॥४०॥

Samāna-jayāt-jvalanam||40||

By mastering (jayāt) Samāna -one of the five vital forces (samāna), effulgence, radiance or divine glow (jvalanam) is attained ||40||

Mastery over samāna brings effulgence, or radiance. Samana vayu is one of the panch-pranas or vital life forces and is believed to reside in the abdomen with the navel as its energy centre. This regulates the digestion of food as well as all our mental process.

श्रोत्राकाशयोः सम्बन्धसंयमाद्दिव्यं श्रोत्रम्॥४१॥

Shrotra-akāśayoḥ sambandha-saṁyamāt-divyaṁ shrotram||41||

Through Saṁyama (saṁyamāt) on the connection or relation (sambandha) between the power of hearing (shrotra) *and* the space or void (ākāśayoḥ), divine (divyam) Power of Hearing (shrotram) *is attained*||41||

By mastering samyama between akasha -space or ether and the power of hearing, one attains the higher, or divine power of hearing. Here Sadhaka will hear divine sounds or seed mantras of chakras, aum, or OM, etc.

कायाकाशयोः सम्बन्धसंयमाल्लघुतूलसमापत्तेश्चाकाशगमनम्॥४२॥

Kāya-akāshayoḥ sambandha-saṁyamāt-laghu-tūla-samāpatteh-cha-akāsha-gamanam||42||

By mastering Saṁyama (saṁyamāt) on the relationship (sambandha) between the physical body (kāya) *and the space, ether or void* (ākāśayoḥ); and (cha) by Samadhi or union (samāpatteḥ) into the subtle or small (laghu) light like cotton (tūla), movement (gamanam) through the space (ākāśa) is acquired||42||

By Samyama on the relationship between the body and space (akasha) one can become so small and light like cotton thread and can travel the space.

वहिरकल्पिता वृत्तिर्महाविदेहा ततः प्रकाशावरणक्षयः ॥४३॥

Bahira-akalpitā vṛittih-mahā-videhā tataḥ prakāsha-avaraṇa-kṣayaḥ||43||

A unimagined (akalpitā) concept or idea (vṛittiḥ) *which is* outside of our experience (bahir), is the great (mahā) formless (videhā). That great and formless (tatas), removes or clears (kṣayaḥ) of the veil or covering (āvaraṇa) over the Inner Light (prakāśa)||43||

When the formless thought patterns of the mind are focussed outside the body, which is known as maha-videha, the great one beyond the body. By samyama on that outward projection, the covering on the spiritual light is removed.

स्थूलस्वरूपसूक्ष्मान्वयार्थवत्त्वसंयमाद्भूतजयः ॥४४॥

Sthūla-svarūpa-sūkṣma-anvaya-arthavattva-saṁyamāt-bhūta-jayaḥ||44||

Through mastering Saṁyama (saṁyamāt) on the gross (sthūla), it's essential nature (sva-rūpa), subtleness (sūkṣma), inherent qualities (anvaya) objectiveness or meaningfulness (arthavattva) of the five Elements (bhūta) one masters those Elements (jayaḥ) ||44||

By samyama on the Bhutas or elements in the form of their gross form, essence, subtleness, inter-relations, and its purpose, one gains mastery over those bhutas.

ततोऽणिमादिप्रादुर्भावः
कायसम्पत्तद्धर्मानभिघातश्च ॥४५॥

Tatas-aṇimā-adi-prādurbhāvaḥ kaya-sampad-tad-dharma-anabhighātash-cha||45||

From the above Samyama (tatas), *there are* fruits (prādurbhāvaḥ) of the supernormal power of minimization (aṇimā), etc. (ādi), of body (kāya) is perfected (sampad) and (cha) non-obstruction or freedom (anabhighātaḥ) in respect of the physical characteristics (dharma) of that *body* (tad)||45||

Through that mastery over the elements, one achieves the ability of making the body atomically small, perfect, and indestructible in its characteristics or components, as well as such other powers. Also it can be seen as being free of our own bodily characteristics and of biological forces causing desires, which result in chitta-vrittis.

रूपलावण्यबलवज्रसंहननत्वानि कायसम्पत् ॥४६॥

Rūpa-lāvaṇya-bala-vajra-saṁhananatvāni kaya-sampat||46||

Bodily (kāya) mastery (sampad) *in form of* beauty (rūpa), charm (lāvaṇya), strength (bala) vitality (vajra) and solidity is attained (saṁhananatvāni)||46||

This mastery of the body brings beauty, gracefulness, strength, and adamantine, vitality and solidity in bearing challenges that come.

ग्रहणस्वरूपास्मितान्वयार्थवत्त्वसंयमादिन्द्रियजयः ॥४७॥
Grahaṇa-svarūpa-asmitā-anvaya-arthavattva-saṁyamāt-indriya-jayaḥ||47||

Through practise of Saṁyama (saṁyamāt) on perception (grahaṇa), essential nature (sva-rūpa), I-ness (asmitā), inherence (anvaya) *meaningfulness* (arthavattva) *one masters* (jayaḥ) the sensory organs (indriya)||47||

By samyama on the process of receiving and perceiving, and it's essence, I-ness, inter-relations, and purpose of senses and their acts, one gains mastery over those senses and their acts (indriyas).

ततो मनोजवित्वं विकरणभावः प्रधानजयश्च ॥४८॥
Tato manas-javitvaṁ vikaraṇa-bhāvaḥ pradhāna-jayash-cha||48||

From the above *Saṁyama* (tatas), sharpness of skilfulness (javitvam) of the mind (manas), a state (bhāvaḥ) in which the sensory organs act independently of the body and mind (vikaraṇa), and (cha) mastery (jayaḥ) over the Prakriti or Mother Nature is attained (pradhāna)||48||

By that mastery over the senses and their acts (indriyas), one attains attentiveness of mind, and perception through the senses becomes free from our body-mind influences. Here further one gains mastery or knowledge of the primal cause of manifestation. Prakriti is known as mother nature or the primary source of every thing that exists or manifests.

सत्त्वपुरुषान्यताख्यातिमात्रस्य सर्वभावाधिष्ठातृत्वं सर्वज्ञातृत्वं च॥४९॥

Sattva-puruṣa-anyatā-khyāti-mātrasya sarva-bhāva-adhiṣṭhātṛatvaṁ sarva-jñātṛatvaṁ cha||49||

The one who is well established in discriminative knowledge or viveka (khyāti-mātrasya) of the difference (anyatā) between pure intellect (sattva) *and* Self (puruṣa), it brings supremacy or mastery (adhiṣṭhātṛtvam) over all (sarvand) beings or that exist (bhāva) and (hca) omniscience, those beyond existence (sarvajñātṛtvam)||49||

To one who has mastered the knowledge of the distinction between the purest aspect of the mind and consciousness or puruṣa itself and the discriminative intellect or viveka, one attains supremacy over all forms or states of existence, as well as over all forms of knowing which is beyond material existence or experience.

तद्वैराग्यादपि दोषवीजक्षये कैवल्यम्॥५०॥

Tad-vairājnāt-api doṣa-bīja-kṣaye kaivalyam||50||

By mastering detachment (vairājnāt) even (api) of that Viveka (tad), there is removal or purification (kṣaye) of the seeds (bīja) of impurities (doṣa), Liberation or Self-Realisation (kaivalyam) is attained||50||

With non-attachment for that supremacy over forms and states of existence and the omniscience is mastered, the seeds at the root of all the bondages are destroyed, and absolute liberation is attained.

स्थान्युपनिमन्त्रणे सङ्गस्मयाकरणं
पुनरनिष्टप्रसङ्गात्॥५१॥

Sthāni-upanimantraṇe saṅga-smaya-akaraṇaṁ punar-aniṣṭa-prasaṅgāt||51||

When invited (upanimantraṇe) by celestial beings (sthāni), *one* should not accept that (saṅga- akaraṇam) nor should it be allowed to cause (akaraṇam) conceit, pride or ego (smaya), since it has the possibility (prasaṅgāt) of undesirable results (punar-aniṣṭa)||51||

When invited by the celestial beings, one should not allow either acceptance or pride in them, because if one allows such thoughts to arise again, it will create the possibility of repeating undesirable thoughts, actions and fruits.

क्षणतत्क्रमयोः संयमाद्विवेकजं ज्ञानम्॥५२॥

Kṣaṇa-tat-kramayoḥ saṁyamāt-viveka-jaṁ jñānam||52||

Through Saṁyama (saṁyamāt) on moment (kṣaṇa) *and* its (tad) sequence or order (kramayoḥ), a knowledge (jñānam) which arises (jam) from discrimination (viveka)is attained ||52||

By samyama on the moments and their sequence or series, one achieves the higher knowledge that is born from discrimination.

जातिलक्षणदेशैरन्यतानवच्छेदात्तुल्ययोस्ततः
प्रतिपत्तिः ॥५३॥

Jāti-lakṣaṇa-deshaih-anyatā-anavacchedāt-tulyayoh-tataḥ pratipattiḥ||53||

From that *knowledge* (tatas), there is clear perception *or the knowledge of difference* (pratipattiḥ) between two things which are alike (tulyayoḥ) even though difference (anyatā) is indescribable (anavacchedāt) by means of class or species (jāti), basic character (lakṣaṇa) and position or place (deshaiḥ)||53||

From that discriminative wisdom one masters awareness of the distinction between two similar objects, which are otherwise not distinguishable by category, characteristics, or position in the universe. The Yogī can perceive or experience the difference through that Viveka, knowledge obtained by practicing Saṁyama on changes and its sequence.

तारकं सर्वविषयं सर्वथाविषयमक्रमं चेति विवेकजं ज्ञानम्॥५४॥

Tārakaṁ sarva-viṣayaṁ sarvathā-viṣayam-akramaṁ ch-eti viveka-jaṁ jñānam||54||

Knowledge (jñānam) which arises (jam) from discrimination (viveka) is intuitive or transcendental knowledge (tārakam). *Which is* comprehensive of all (sarva) objects and their subjects (viṣayam) manifesting (viṣayam) at all times (sarvathā) and (cha) has no sequence (akramam... iti)||54||

That higher knowledge is intuitive and transcendent, and is rooted and acquired of discrimination; it includes all objects and conditions related to them within their field, and is beyond any sequences.

सत्त्वपुरुषयोः शुद्धिसाम्ये कैवल्यमिति॥५५॥

Sattva-puruṣayoḥ shuddhi-sāmye kaivalyam-iti||55||

When there is equality or union (sāmye) of purity (shuddhi) and purest consciousness (sattva) *and* divine Self or Atman (puruṣayoḥ), the state of highest liberation or emancipation (kaivalyam iti) *manifests* ||55||

With the attainment of union between the purest aspect the mind, chitta and buddhi and the pure consciousness, purusha, or soul, one achieves liberation, or enlightenment and that is the end goal.

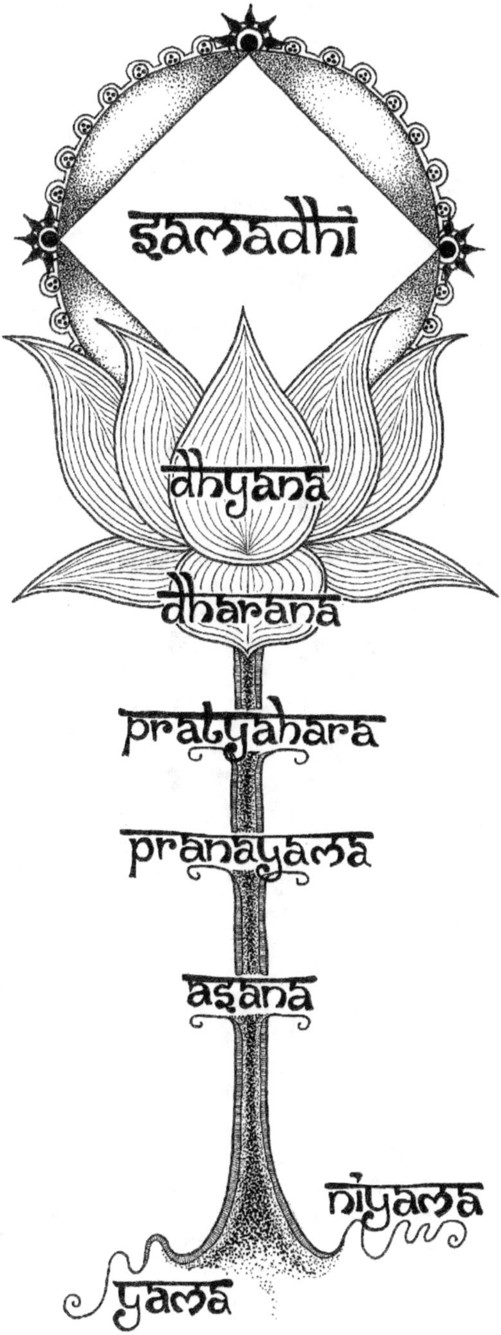
samadhi
dhyana
dharana
pratyahara
pranayama
asana
niyama
yama

Chapter 4 : Kaivalya Pāda

जन्मौषधिमन्त्रतपःसमाधिजाः सिद्धयः॥१॥
Janma-uṣadhi-mantra-tapaḥ-samādhi-jāḥ siddhayaḥ||1||

The Siddhis or Supernatural
Powers (siddhayaḥ) come (jāḥ) with birth (janma), *or can be attained by* herbs (auṣadhi), mantras (mantra), austerities, sadhana or practise (tapas) *self-realisation or union* (samādhi)||1||

Those Siddhis, supernatural powers or transcendental awareness is attained by birth or can be attained through herbs, mantra, austerities, and union through meditation.

जात्यन्तरपरिणामः प्रकृत्यापूरात्॥२॥
Jātyantarapariṇāmaḥ prakṛtyāpūrāt||2||

The results or transformation (pariṇāmaḥ) into other (antara) births or species (jāti) *is attained* through absorbing awareness in (āpūrāt) their essential nature (prakṛti)||2||

Attainment or transformation into another form or type of birth takes place through the fulfilling of their innate nature. This refers to the power we have to chose the brith through moulding our conscious mind into all the essential nature of that species. This will create the ideal situation for attaining that particular body and life. This is like using our skills to mould the clay into any shape we like.

निमित्तमप्रयोजकं प्रकृतीनां वरणभेदस्तु ततः क्षेत्रिकवत् ॥३॥

Nimittam-aprayojakaṁ prakṛatīnāṁ varaṇa-bhedah-tu tataḥ kṣetrika-vat||3||

Action or accidental cause (nimittam) *does not bring* the essential natures (prakṛtīnām) into motion, which are not brought into action (aprayojakam) but (tu) it removes (bhedaḥ) the obstacles (varaṇa). For that reason (tatas), it is like (vat) the farmer (kṣetrika) (*who removes a barrier or mound so that the water can flow to irrigate his crops)* ||3||

Actions and practices done incidentally do not bring experiences, attainment or realisations. One achieves realisations by removing obstacles and disturbances.

Its like irrigating your garden or vegetation, you will need to open and run the tap or allow the water to flow and not just direct the hose around your vegetation. Or if you want to enjoy the heat of the fire, you will need to put effort into lighting the fire and not just sit around the fire pit and wait for the heat.

निर्माणचित्तान्यस्मितामात्रात् ॥४॥

Nirmāṇa-chittān—asmitā-mātrāt||4||

The emerging or arising (nirmāṇa) experiences of the mind (chittāni) are *produced* from only or alone (mātrāt) I-ness (asmitā)||4||

The perception or experience of mind fields comes from the individuality of I-ness (asmita). Here Patanjali explains that what we see, hear, feel, taste, all those experiences are arising under the influence of I-ness of liking-disliking, pain-pleasure based on past experiences.

प्रवृत्तिभेदे प्रयोजकं चित्तमेकमनेकेषाम्॥५॥
Pravṛitti-bhede prayojakaṁ chittam-ekam-anekeṣām||5||

One (ekam) mind (chittam) *brings forth* the many *minds* (anekeṣām) into action (prayojakam) during their different and divergent (bhede) activities (pravṛtti)||5||

From the One conscious mind, due to different or divergent adverse activities of the mind fields, many other minds are produces or taking place from the One Conscious mind. Here the Pure Conscious Mind is the source of all other minds arising from it due to various adverse activities.

तत्र ध्यानजमनाशयम्॥६॥
Tatra dhyāna-jam-anāshayam||6||

Of these *arising minds* (tatra), brought about (jam) through meditation (dhyāna) are free of any (an) latent impressions (āshayam)||6||

Of these many mind fields, the one that has emerged and grown from meditation is free from any latent impressions produced from karma or actions.

कर्माशुक्लाकृष्णं योगिनस्त्रिविधमितरेषाम् ॥७॥
Karma-ashukla-akṛaṣṇaṁ yoginah-trividham-itareṣām||7||

The actions (karma) of a Yogī (yoginaḥ) are neither uncoloured (ashukla) nor coloured (akṛṣṇam), *while* Karmas of others (itareṣām) are of three types (trividham)||7||

The actions or karmas of yogis are neither coloured or uncoloured and produce no impressions. While the Karma and their results are of three types for others.

ततस्तद्विपाकानुगुणानामेवाभिव्यक्तिर्वासनानाम् ॥८॥
Tatas-tad-vipāka-anuguṇānām-eva-abhivyaktih-vāsanānām||8||

From those three kinds of actions (tatas), *there is* certainly (eva) manifestation or result (abhivyaktiḥ) of latent impressions or potential seeds (vāsanānām) following or corresponding (anuguṇānām) to the consequences or results (vipāka) of those three types of Karma(tad)||8||

Those threefold actions or karmas result in deep rooted latent impressions (**vāsanā**) that will later come to fruition corresponding to those karmic impressions. **Vāsanās are latent impressions or potential seeds which are produced by birth, life-span and experience of pleasure and pain.**

जातिदेशकालव्यवहितानामप्यानन्तर्यं
स्मृतिसंस्कारयोरेकरूपत्वात्॥९॥

Jāti-desha-kāla-vyavahitānām-api-ānantaryaṁ smṛiti-saṁskārayoh-ekarūpatvāt||9||

Because of similarity in form (ekarūpatvāt) between memory (smṛiti) *and* samskara or latent impressions (saṁskārayoḥ), *there is* uninterrupted sequence (ānantaryam) *of* vāsanā even though (api) in between or gap (vyavahitānām) by birth (jāti), space or place (desha) *and* time (kāla)||9||

Smriti or memory and samaskaras or the deep habit patterns seems to be the same in appearance. There is always an uninterrupted sequence in between those traits, even though there might be different location, time, or state of life. This Sutra explains that that as long as there are vāsanā, smṛiti, and saṁskāra, there will always be an uninterrupted sequence between all those, Karma and their fruits.

तासामनादित्वं चाशिषो नित्यत्वात्॥१०॥

Tāsām-anāditvaṁ cha-āshiṣah nityatvāt||10||

The desire for life (āśiṣaḥ) is eternal (nityatvāt), those *Vāsanās* (tāsām) *from where they arise* also (cha) has no beginning (anāditvam)||10||

These samaskaras and *Vāsanās* have no beginning to their processes due to the eternal and continuous nature of the desire to live.

हेतुफलाश्रयालम्बनैः सङ्गृहीतत्वादेषामभावे तदभावः॥११॥

Hetu-phala-āshraya-ālambanaiḥ saṅgṛhītatvāt-eṣām-abhāve tad-abhāvaḥ||11||

Since *Vāsanās* are held in us together (saṅgṛhītatvāt) by cause (hetu), fruit or result (phala), dependence or refuge (āśraya) *and* support of the objects (ālambanaiḥ), in the absence (abhāve) of those above (cause, fruit or result, dependence and support) (eṣām), *there comes* absence (abhāvaḥ) of those *vāsanās* (tad)||11||

Vāsanās are accumulated and held in us together by cause, fruit or motive, object dependence. These all disappear when *Vāsanās* are removed or let go.

अतीतानागतं स्वरूपतोऽस्त्यध्वभेदाद्धर्माणाम्॥१२॥

Atīta-anāgataṁ svarūpatah-asti-adhva-bhedāt-dharmāṇām||12||

Past (atīta) *and* future (anāgatam) *Vāsanās* exist (asti) in their essential forms (sva-rūpataḥ). *The only difference* is in the characteristics of the forms (dharmāṇām) at different (bhedāt) times or phases like past, present, and future (adhva)||12||

Past and future samaskaras and *Vāsanās* exist in the present as if they are real, but they appear differently because of their different characteristics or forms regarding the time or phases as past, present and future.

ते व्यक्तसूक्ष्मा गुणात्मानः ॥१३॥

Te vyakta-sūkṣmā guṇa-ātmānaḥ||13||

Those *characteristics* (te) are manifest or experienced (vyakta) *and* are subtle (sūkṣmāḥ) *and* contain (ātmānaḥ) their *three* Guṇās (guṇ)||13||

These samaskaras, and *Vāsanās*, their characteristics and forms, manifested, experienced or subtle, they are composed of three primary Gunas or qualities. These three qualities are Sattva, Rajas and Tamas.

परिणामैकत्वाद्वस्तुतत्त्वम् ॥१४॥

Pariṇāma-ekatvāt-vastu-tattvam||14||

Due to the oneness or uniformity (ekatvāt) results of the three Gunās (pariṇāma), an object (vastu) appears to be real (tattvam)||14||

The characteristics of an object appear as a single unit, of the oneness and uniformity due to the reason they manifested from their primary qualities. Due to this appearance the objects or their experiences seem to be as if they are real.

वस्तुसाम्ये चित्तभेदात्तयोर्विभक्तः पन्थाः॥१५॥

Vastu-sāmye chitta-bhedāt-tayoh-vibhaktaḥ panthāḥ||15||

Despite oneness (sāmye) of objects (vastu), there is a different (vibhaktaḥ) ways of perceiving (panthāḥ) to both of them (the object and their inherited qualities) (tayoḥ) due to different (bhedāt) minds (chitta)||15||

The same objects are perceived differently by different minds as each mind perceives them in different ways depending on their own manifestation and conditioning.

Same life situations or events will be perceived differently by different people. This depends on our personal mind and our family, social and cultural conditioning or training.

न चैकचित्ततन्त्रं वस्तु तदप्रमाणकं तदा किं स्यात्॥१६॥

Na chaika-chitta-tantraṁ vastu tad-apramāṇakaṁ tadā kiṁ syāt||16||

The object (vastu) certainly (cha) is not (na) dependent (tantram) on only one (eka) mind (chitta), *because of* what (kim) would happen (syāt) when *it* is not experienced or known (apramāṇakam) by the mind (tad) then (tadā)?||16||

However, the object and its reality is independent of any of these minds. If It was not, then what will happen to the object if it is not being experienced by that mind? So all the objects of experiences are free or un-effected by our perception.

तदुपरागापेक्षित्वाच्चित्तस्य वस्तु ज्ञाताज्ञातम् ॥१७॥
Tad-uparāga-apekṣitvāt-chittasya vastu jñāta-ajñātam||17||

The object (vastu) is known (jñāta) *or* unknown (ajñātam) to the mind (chittasya) according to how (apekṣitvāt) it colours (uparāga) that *mind* (tad)||17||

Objects are either known or not known depending of the conditioning or colouring of the mind perceiving that object. If that object did not leave any impression or did not attract our attention, even if it is there, we would not know it. Also our knowledge or experience will be the outcome of how we perceive it.

सदा ज्ञाताश्चित्तवृत्तयस्तत्प्रभोः पुरुषस्यापरिणामित्वात् ॥१८॥
Sadā jñātāh-chitta-vṛittayah-tat-prabhoḥ puruṣasyā-pariṇāmitvāt||18||

To the Divine or Higher Consciousness (prabhoḥ) of the mind (tad), the mental (chitta) modifications or whirlpools (vṛittayaḥ) *are* always (sadā) known (jñātāḥ) because permanent or non-changeable (apariṇāmitvāt) nature of Self or Atman (puruṣasya)||18||

The whirlpools of the mind are always known by the awareness or pure consciousness. Pure consciousness is superior, and it masters the mundane mind.

न तत्स्वाभासं दृश्यत्वात् ॥१९॥

Na tat-sva-ābhāsaṁ dṛashyatvāt||19||

That *mind* (tad) is not (na) self-illuminating (sva-ābhāsam) as it is a knowable or manifested object (dṛashyatvāt)||19||

That mind is the manifest object of the knowledge and perception of pure consciousness. Hence the mind is not independently self illuminating.

एकसमये चोभयानवधारणम् ॥२०॥

Ekasamaye cha-ubhaya-anava-dhāraṇam||20||

And (cha) there is no knowing or experience (anava-dhāraṇam) of them both (mind and objects of experience) (ubhaya) at one time (ekasamaye)||20||

At one point either the mind or the illuminating process can be cognised or perceived. The both factors cannot be perceived simultaneously or at the same time.

चित्तान्तरदृश्ये बुद्धिबुद्धेरतिप्रसङ्गः
स्मृतिसङ्करश्च ॥२१॥

Chitta-antara-dṛashye buddhi-buddheh-atiprasaṅgaḥ smṛati-saṅkarash-cha||21||

If the mind is a knowable object (dṛashye) to another (antara) mind (chitta), *then there would be endless events* (atiprasaṅgaḥ) of wisdom of Knower (buddheḥ-buddhi) and (cha) confusion or intermixture (saṅkaraḥ) of memories (smṛati)||21||

If one mind is manifested from another, as the first one from master (pure consciousness), then there would be endless events or perceptions, or cognition and confusion if the mind is an object to be known.

This is our modern mind, manifesting from multitasking personalities. We are trying to do too many things at once. Listening, watching, reading, and doing various things along with all the mental dialogues going on. It illuminates minds from the mind and we lose our energy, integrity, balance and mindfulness.

चितेरप्रतिसङ्क्रमायास्तदाकारापत्तौ स्वबुद्धिसंवेदनम् ॥२२॥

Chiteh-apratisaṅkramāyāh-tad-ākāra-āpattau sva-buddhi-saṁvedanam||22||

When Consciousness (chiteḥ), though non-changing or permanent (apratisaṅkramāyāḥ), assumed or transformed into (āpattau) the form (ākāra) of the Buddhi (tad), *it identifies or experiences* (saṁvedanam) one's own Self (sva) and Buddhi (buddhi)||22||

When the non-changing consciousness takes form or transforms into that finest aspect of the conscious mind, then one experiences or perceives process of one's own perception. This is knowing the process or knowing itself.

द्रष्टृदृश्योपरक्तं चित्तं सर्वार्थम् ॥२३॥

Draṣṭṛa-dṛashya-uparaktaṁ chittaṁ sarva-artham||23||

Mind (chittam), coloured or being effected (uparaktam) by the seer (draṣṭṛa) and the seen (dṛashya), *is* all-comprehensive (sarva-artham)||23||

The conscious mind, which is coloured and conditioned by both seer and seen, has the potential to perceive any and all objects.

तदसङ्ख्येयवासनाभिश्चित्रमपि परार्थं संहत्यकारित्वात्॥२४॥

Tad-asaṅkhyeya-vāsanābhih-chitram-api parārthaṁ saṁhatya-kāritvāt||24||

The *mind* (tad), although (api) exhibiting various colors (chitram) by countless (asaṅkhyeya) vāsanās not in action (vāsanābhiḥ), *exists* for another meaning (para-artham) as it is in action (kāritvāt) in combination (saṁhatya)||24||

That conscious mind field is filled with countless impressions and **vāsanās**. It exists as witnessing consciousness, as the mind field is operating only in combination with those impressions or **vāsanās**.

विशेषदर्शिन आत्मभावभावनाविनिवृत्तिः॥२५॥

Visheṣa-darshina ātma-bhāva-bhāvanā-vinivṛattiḥ||25||

To one who have experienced (darshinaḥ) the special distinction (visheṣa) (in Self or Knower and what is to be known) there is complete cessation (vinivṛattiḥ) of the feelings and deep thoughts (bhāvanā) in the nature (bhāva) of his own Self (ātma)||25||

Once Sadhaka has experienced the distinction between awareness or seer and the subtlest mind, Sadhaka will not have false perceptions, not even at the level of deep thoughts or feelings.

तदा विवेकनिम्नङ्कैवल्यप्राग्भारञ्चित्तम् ॥२६॥

Tadā viveka-nimnam-kaivalya-prāk-bhāram-chittam||26||

Then (tadā), the mind (chittam) inclines or drawn (nimnam) towards discriminative *knowledge* (viveka) *and* is directed (prāk-bhāram) toward Absolute Liberation (kaivalya)||26||

Then the conscious mind is drawn towards the highest discriminatory wisdom or knowledge (viveka), and it is naturally drawn or inclined to attain Absolute Liberation.

तच्छिद्रेषु प्रत्ययान्तराणि संस्कारेभ्यः ॥२७॥

Tad-chidreṣu pratyaya-antarāṇi saṁskārebhyaḥ||27||

In between the gaps or intervals (chidreṣu) of the Viveka (tad), other (antarāṇi) mental modifications, cause or contents (pratyaya) *rise from deep and subtle* impressions (saṁskārebhyaḥ)||27||

In between the gaps in those higher discriminative wisdom or viveka, other deep rooted samskaras or thought patterns and impressions arise from the unconscious mind.

हानमेषां क्लेशवदुक्तम् ॥२८॥
Hānam-eṣāṁ klesha-vat-uktam||28||

It is said (uktam) *that* the removal (hānam) of the mental modifications (eṣām) similar to (vat) the Klesha or Afflictions (klesha)||28||

To remove these samskaras interfering, we use the same processes or tools as being described previously to deal with colouring or states of mind as Pancha-Kleshas.

प्रसङ्ख्यानेऽप्यकुसीदस्य सर्वथा विवेकख्यातेर्धर्ममेघः समाधिः ॥२९॥
Prasaṅkhyāne-api-akusīdasya sarvathā viveka-khyāter-dharma-meghaḥ samādhiḥ||29||

Once attained discriminative wisdom (viveka-khyāteḥ) in the highest form and at all times (sarvathā), does not take an interest (akusīdasya) even (api) in *that* omniscience resulting from Discriminatory Wisdom (prasaṅkhyāne), Samādhi or Perfect Absorption in Meditation (samādhiḥ) *known as* Dharma-megha or Abundance of Virtue occurs (dharma-meghaḥ)||29||

With discrimination, when one even have no interest in the highest wisdom, Samadhi occurs. This brings an abundance of virtues, reasoning and discrimination. The Highest Samadhi occurs when yogic even let go the desire to be liberated. As long as there are any Samaskaras or Vasanas even of enlightenment, there will be series of desires, thoughts and actions. Highest Samadhi occurs once we completely let go of our mind-field, I-ness, and desires.

ततः क्लेशकर्मनिवृत्तिः ॥३०॥
Tataḥ klesha-karma-nivṛttiḥ||30||

From the Dharma-megha Samadhi (tatas),
there is cessation (nivṛttiḥ) of
Afflictions (klesha) *and* actions (karma)||30||

With this Dharma-Megha Samadhi, kleshas or colouring of the mind and Karmic bondages are removed or purified.

तदा सर्वावरणमलापेतस्य ज्ञानस्यानन्त्याज्ज्ञेयमल्पम् ॥३१॥
Tadā sarva-āvaraṇa-mala-apetasya jñānasya-ānantyāt-jñeyam-alpam||31||

Then (tadā), due to the infinite (ānantyāt)
knowledge (jñānasya) removal (apetasya) of
all (sarva) layers or coverings (āvaraṇa) of
impurities (mala), the what to know (jñeyam) *is almost nothing* (alpam)||31||

Once those kleshas and karmas are removed, one experiences the Infinite. Here one attains the highest realisation where nothing is to be known anymore. This is the state of all-knowing or Divine-Realisation, where nothing else is to be known anymore.

ततः कृतार्थानां परिणामक्रमसमाप्तिर्गुणानाम् ॥३२॥

Tataḥ kṛata-arthānāṁ pariṇāma-krama-samāptih-guṇānām||32||

From the *Dharmamegha Samādhi* (tatas), when the Guṇās (guṇānām) have fulfilled their purpose (kṛata-arthānām), there is cessation or end (samāptiḥ) of the sequence of results (pariṇāma-krama) *of those Gun*ās ||32||

With attainment of this Highest Samadhi, the three primary Gunas (qualities) will have fulfilled their purpose and will not transform into further mixed gunas or qualities. Here they merge back into their primary essence. There will be no further sequence or order of their results, and actions.

क्षणप्रतियोगी परिणामापरान्तनिर्ग्राह्यः क्रमः ॥३३॥

Kṣaṇapratiyogī pariṇāmāparāntanirgrāhyaḥ kramaḥ||33||

Sequence or order (kramaḥ) is of uninterrupted succession (pratiyogī) to the moments (kṣaṇa) *and* is perceivable, recognizable, apprehensible (nirgrāhyaḥ) at the termination (aparānta) of the results or fruits (pariṇāma)||33||

The sequencing or ordering process which is uninterrupted succession of moments and impressions corresponds to the time, and is recognisable at the end point of the sequence.

पुरुषार्थशून्यानां गुणानां प्रतिप्रसवः कैवल्यं
स्वरूपप्रतिष्ठा वा चितिशक्तिरिति ॥३४॥

Puruṣa-artha-shūnyānāṁ guṇānāṁ pratiprasavaḥ
kaivalyaṁ sva-rūpa-pratiṣṭhā vā chiti-shaktih-iti||34||

Absolute Liberation (kaivalyam) or (vā) the Power (shaktiḥ) of Consciousness (chiti) established (pratiṣṭhā) in her own nature (sva-rūpa) *occurs when* the Guṇas (guṇānām) merge back into their source (pratiprasavaḥ), as they have no *more* purpose to fulfil (artha-shūnyānām) for Puruṣa (puruṣa) is The End (iti) ||34||

When those primary qualities or elements merge back or resolve back into the source they emerged from. This brings the highest or absolute liberation, here pure consciousness becomes established in its own TRUE NATURE.

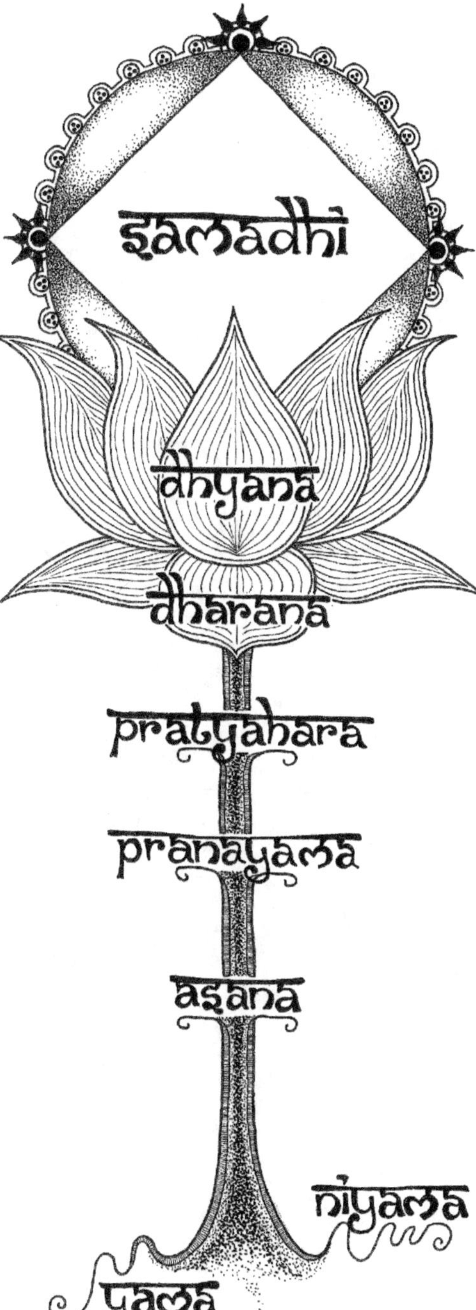
samadhi
dhyana
dharana
pratyahara
pranayama
asana
niyama
yama

www.ingramcontent.com/pod-product-compliance
Lightning Source LLC
Chambersburg PA
CBHW071247070526
44583CB00017B/2356
9781999585037